Phenotypic Oncology PET

Ching Yee Oliver Wong • Dafang Wu

Phenotypic Oncology PET

An Instructional Casebook

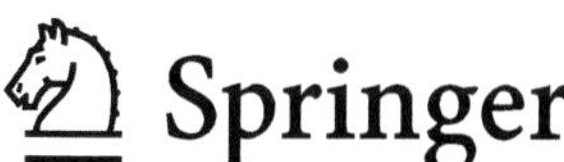

Springer

Ching Yee Oliver Wong
Sutter Health Imaging
Sacramento, CA, USA

Dafang Wu
Northern California PET Imaging Center
Sacramento, CA, USA

ISBN 978-3-031-09739-3   ISBN 978-3-031-09737-9   (eBook)
https://doi.org/10.1007/978-3-031-09737-9

This Springer imprint is published by the registered company Springer Nature Switzerland AG
The registered company address is: Gewerbestrasse 11, 6330 Cham, Switzerland

Preface

PET is a molecular imaging tool for oncologic applications. The PET tracers depict the tumor phenotypes for diagnostic evaluation and cellular population changes after therapy. Therefore, there are no biological false-negative PET scans. Each tumor expresses a wide spectrum of tracer uptake in the same individual or among different patients. For instance, a low-grade lymphoma usually has a lower uptake in F-18 FDG PET than that of a high-grade lymphoma reflecting different phenotypes. The same size of tumor can produce a different uptake in many PET tracers. In lung cancer, these PET phenotypes are more useful than the uniformly high FDG uptake. In case of growing lung nodule, it is highly suspicious of malignancy. Different uptake in PET, even no uptake (subjected to physical limitation of partial volume effects) for the same tumor size can offer additional phenotypic information. The squamous cell, small cell, or sarcomatous lung cancer have usually more uptake in FDG than that of the well-differentiated adenocarcinoma. In neuroendocrine tumor, the FDG uptake is proportional to the grade of tumor while Ga-68 or Cu-64 DOTATATE has a reversed patten. In prostate cancer, FDG is usually low in uptake, but F-18 Fluciclovine or F-18 PSMA has high in uptake. The CT features already provide anatomical tumor information in case of low PET tracer uptake, and there is often no need for uniform high uptake in PET for diagnosis. With modern PET-CT imaging, the reader should place emphasis on PET phenotypes rather than simply positive or negative uptake in PET, especially differential tracers are employed. Some false-positive PET cases are also provided, including recent COVID-19 vaccination. Since there are many PET tracers available for clinical use, the knowledge of potential different PET phenotypes can help the oncologists to select the most appreciate tracer(s) for diagnosis and treatment planning.

After therapy, there are fundamental changes in the cellular population, from tumor cells to fibroblasts or normal cells. The collective information from cellular phenotypes provides the response assessment. Quantification can further assist the PET evaluation which is included in many cases and further supplements the illustration of cellular phenotypes for clinical oncologic applications.

The history and images are presented with questions. The first question for each case always starts with the tracer(s) which the reader can infer from the tracer distribution on the maximum projection image (MIP) of PET. Interpretation and teaching points are presented in the following pages with references. If there are more than one case with same tumor types, different teaching points and references are provided. The reader can use the index to search for certain tumor types or to group them into categories for didactic learning. For those taking board examination or maintenance of certificate (MOC), it may be more challenging to go by the order of the case. For clinical scenario of rare cases, the table of content may serve as a quick reference.

Sacramento, CA, USA   Ching Yee Oliver Wong
Sacramento, CA, USA   Dafang Wu

Acknowledgments

I sincerely thank Dr. Richard H. Kennedy, PhD, Professor and Vice President Research at Beaumont Health, Michigan, USA, for his persistent support and encouragement in this current project and during my prior textbook writing 3 years ago. I need to acknowledge that most of the cases presented in this book were from patients I had been privileged to serve in the Nuclear Medicine Clinic of Beaumont Hospital, Royal Oak, Michigan. This project would not have been possible without their unlimited contribution to medical science and education.

I am deeply grateful to my entire family for their continued support in my scholarly endeavors. Most of all, I wish to thank my wife, Xiaoping, from the bottom of my heart, for her understanding, and for our shared passion in the achievement of best patient care with our best capacities.

Dr. Dafang Wu, MD, PhD

I want to express my greatest gratitude to Dr. Penny Vande Streek, DO, Chief of Nuclear Medicine at Sutter Health, California, USA, for her constant support and encouragement in this current project and during my clinical work on PET-CT imaging over the past 5 years. I am delighted to acknowledge that a lot of cases presented in this book were from patients I had been privileged to serve in the PET-CT imaging of Sutter Health, Sacramento, California This project would not have been possible without the contribution of all staff in Sutter Health Imaging to medical science and education.

I am deeply indebted to the unlimited support of my family for my scholarly endeavors. I wish to thank my daughters Regina and Christiana for their help on the initial word processing; my son William for his advice on image processing; and last but not least my wife Sherry for her understanding of preparing the manuscript days and nights during the COVID-19 pandemic.

Dr. Ching Yee Oliver Wong, MD, PhD

Contents

Chapter 1
Case 1: Double Pulmonary Nodules

A: Baseline PET has standard uptake value (SUV) at right upper lobe (RUL) 15.5 and left upper lobe (LUL) 11.6. (1) What is the tracer? (2) Are the nodules cancerous? (3) Are they double primary or metastasis from each other?

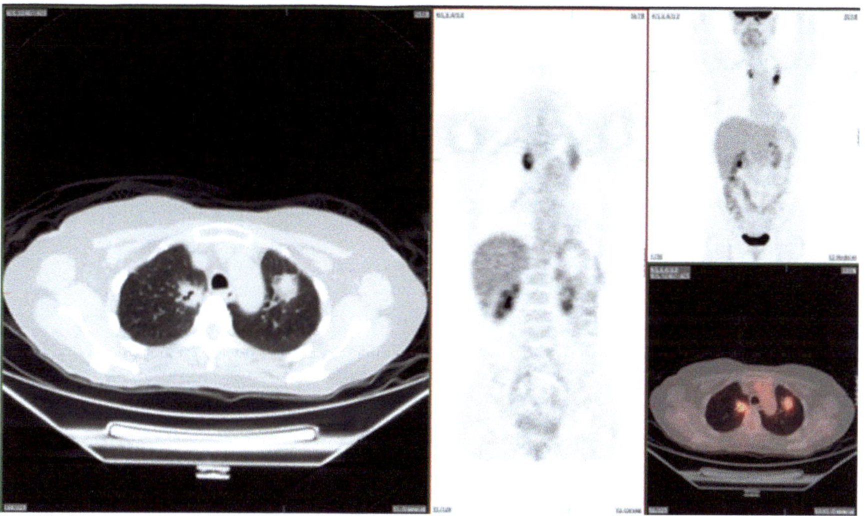

© The Author(s), under exclusive license to Springer Nature Switzerland AG 2022
C. Y. O. Wong, D. Wu, *Phenotypic Oncology PET*,
https://doi.org/10.1007/978-3-031-09737-9_1

B: First-cycle (left and middle panels) and second-cycle (right panel, [SUV]) chemotherapy PET showed SUV at RUL 8.1 [6.3] and LUL 13.6 [10.7]. (1) What is the stage of lung cancer? (2) What is the relative chemosensitivity? (3) Which one is the primary cancer?

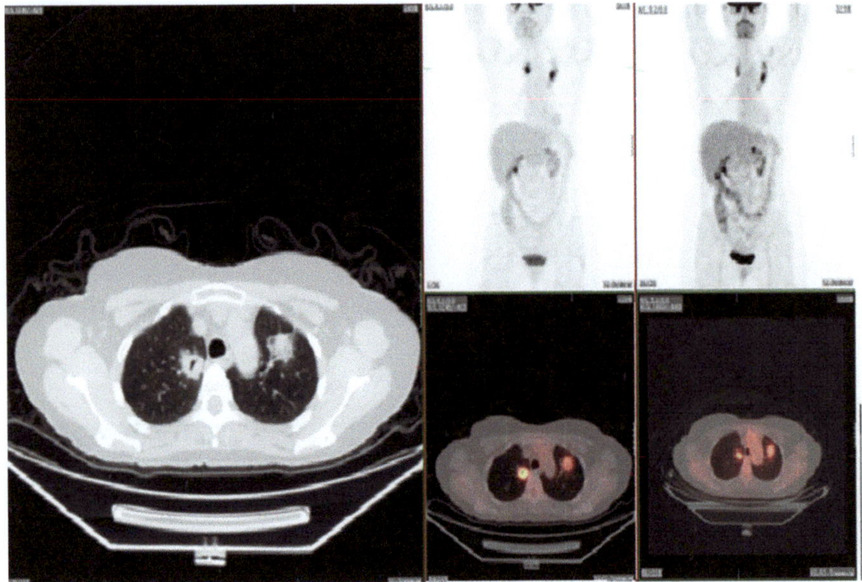

1.1   Case 1: Interpretation and Teaching

A1:   F-18 FDG.
A2:   Focal intense uptake is cancerous until proven otherwise.
A3:   The SUV are so close to each other; they may be the same tumor phenotype.
      But over 50% of the second pulmonary nodule is metastasis.

Pathology RUL core biopsy showed adenocarcinoma, but LUL showed non-small cell lung cancer (NSCLC) with extensive lymphatic invasion. Clonal analysis using colon polyp (as normal tissue control) was performed. DNA isolated from formalin-fixed tissue blocks for polymerase chain reaction (PCR) using primers directed toward common carcinoma mutations revealed identical clones.

B1:   Stage IV from the clonal analysis.
B2:   RUL cancer is more chemosensitive to LUL neoplasm.
B3:   RUL is the primary cancer and LUL is the metastasis.

Teaching Point 1 Metastasis is more resistant than primary cancer. The second-cycle PET showed SUV further decrease at RUL but barely changed at LUL.

Teaching Point 2 Metastasis is the focus of response evaluation.

Reference

Higashiyama M, Okami J, Maeda J, et al. Differences in chemosensitivity between primary and paired metastatic lung cancer tissues: in vitro analysis based on the collagen gel droplet embedded culture drug test (CD-DST). 2012;4(1):40–7.

Chapter 2
Case 2: Nodular Sclerosing Hodgkin's Lymphoma

A: Baseline (leftmost orthogonal panel and first axial and oblique column) as well as two-cycle (middle axial and oblique column) and eight-cycle (third axial and oblique column on rightmost) posttreatment PET in a young female. (1) What is the tracer? (2) What is the distribution pattern of this lymphoma? (3) How is the response?

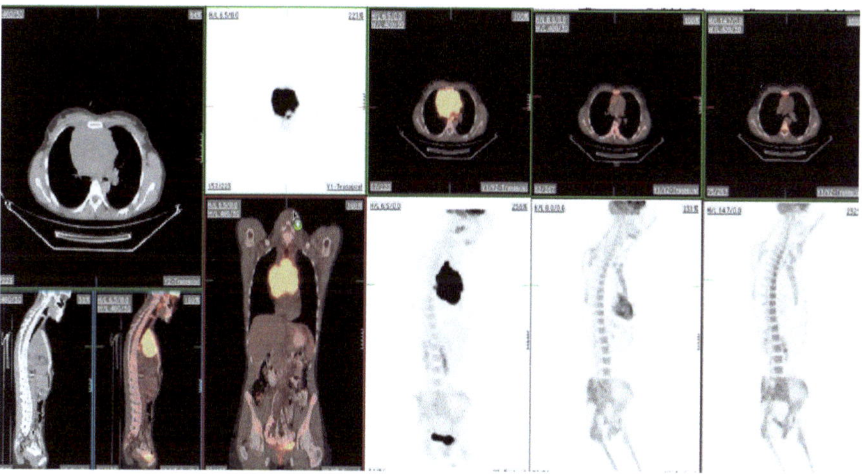

B: Baseline PET showed bulky stage I disease and two-cycle posttreatment PET revealed good chemosensitivity. (1) Why is chemotherapy continued to six cycles? (2) What is the risk of radiation? (3) Is there any hidden bone marrow disease?

C. Y. O. Wong, D. Wu, *Phenotypic Oncology PET*, https://doi.org/10.1007/978-3-031-09737-9_2

2.1 Case 2: Interpretation and Teaching

A1:   F-18 FDG.
A2:   High-grade Hodgkin's lymphoma.
      Teaching point: About 80% Hodgkin's lymphoma is in the chest and mostly in anterior mediastinum. Lymphoma uptake is much higher than liver.
A3:   The patient who received ABVD had a complete response. Deauville 1.

Deauville is a simple tool based on visual interpretation of FDG uptake. It takes advantage of two reference points of the individual patient, which have demonstrated relatively constant uptake on serial imaging. The two reference organs are the blood pool mediastinum (at subcarinal level) and the liver (dome).

The scale ranges from 1 to 5, where 1 is best and 5 is the worst. Each FDG-avid (or previously FDG-avid) lesion is rated independently:

1. No uptake or no residual uptake (when used interim).
2. Slight uptake but equal to or below blood pool (mediastinum).
3. Uptake above mediastinal but below or equal to uptake in the liver.
4. Uptake slightly to moderately higher than liver (less than or equal to twice the maximum).
5. Markedly increased uptake or any new lesion (more than twice the maximum on response evaluation); X for any lesion not overtly attributable to lymphoma.

B1:   There is bulky mediastinal lymphoma which needs consolidative radiation.
B2:   The risk of radiation in a young female is latent effects on breast tissue for a secondary cancer. Thus, reduced dose may be adopted with chemotherapy.
B3:   Since the marrow has generalized augmentation without focal decreased uptake after therapy, there is no metabolic evidence of marrow disease. Bone marrow study showed negative infiltration by aspiration, but it may be subject to sampling error. So when PET show no focal avid foci, marrow aspiration may be omitted in high-grade lymphoma.

2.2   Assessment of Treatment Response

- Complete response (CR): Scores 1, 2, and 3 together with the absence of focally FDG-avid bone marrow lesion(s) are interpreted as complete metabolic response (CR), irrespective of a persistent mass on CT.
- Partial response (PR): A Deauville score of 4 or 5 is provided:

  - Uptake is decreased compared with baseline.
  - Absence of structural progression development on CT.

- Stable disease (SD), also called no metabolic response: A Deauville score of 4 or 5 without significant change in FDG uptake from baseline.
- Progressive disease (PD): A Deauville score of 4–5 with increasing intensity compared to baseline or any interim scan and/or any new FDG-avid focus consistent with malignant lymphoma.

Reference

Hughes-Davies L, Tarbell NJ, Coleman CN, et al. Stage IA-IIB Hodgkin's disease: management and outcome of extensive thoracic involvement. Int J Radiat Oncol Biol Phys. 1997;39:361–9.

Chapter 3
Case 3: Transformation in Non-Hodgkin's Lymphoma

A: Baseline PET in a known grade 1 follicular lymphoma at right inguinal node (SUV 10.6). (1) What is the tracer? (2) Is pathology consistent with PET aggressiveness of the lymphoma?

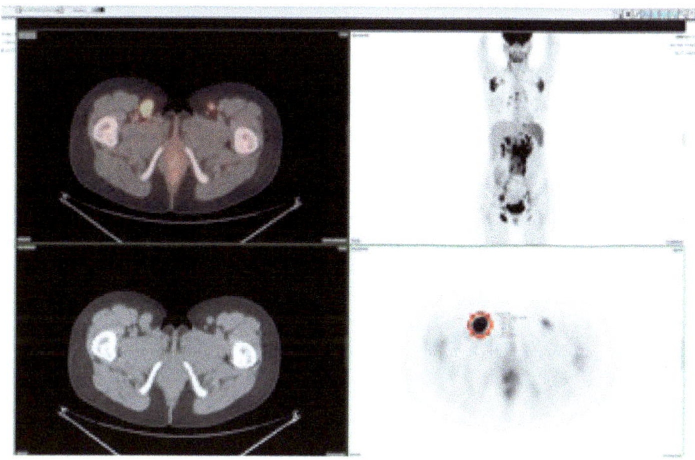

C. Y. O. Wong, D. Wu, *Phenotypic Oncology PET*,
https://doi.org/10.1007/978-3-031-09737-9_3

B: PET 4 months after Rituxan treatment with right inguinal node SUV 7.5 (liver SUV 3.2). (1) What is the response? (2) What is wrong with treatment and/or biopsy?

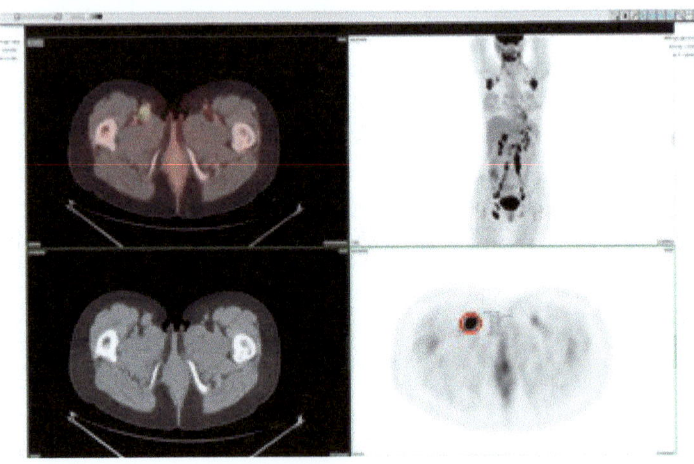

C: PET 11 months after baseline PET with right inguinal node SUV 19.9, but the maximum SUV at the abdomen was 34.1. (1) What is the PET impression of lymphoma? (2) How does PET impact on the treatment?

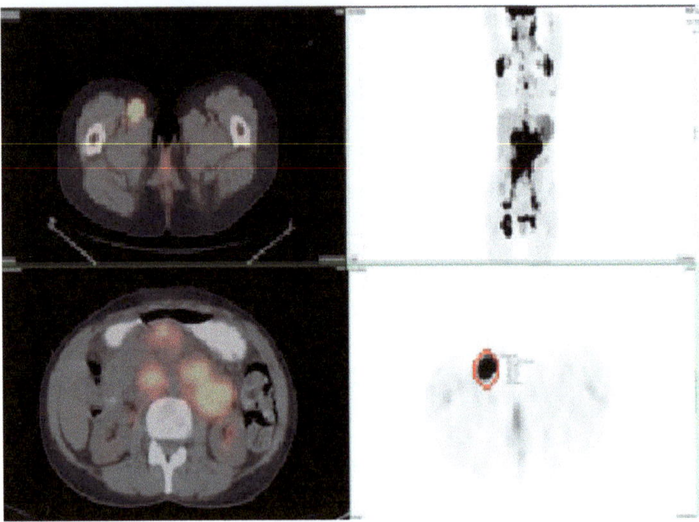

3.1   Case 3: Interpretation and Teaching

A1:   F-18 FDG.
A2:   No. PET indicated an aggressive non-Hodgkin's lymphoma (NHL) inside the abdomen (SUV 34.1).
B1:   The patient who received R-CHOP had a poor response. Deauville 5.
B2:   Treatment was directed at low-grade lymphoma from inguinal node biopsy.

Teaching Point 1   The higher the metabolic uptake, the more aggressive the lymphoma. Biopsy may have a sampling error or not been from highest-grade lymphoma.

C1:   There is likely a transformation of lymphoma. Re-biopsy at the right inguinal node showed diffuse large B-cell lymphoma (DLBCL).
C2:   Treatment was changed for a high-grade lymphoma.

PET after two cycles of R-CHOP: SUV = 2.8 (mediastinal SUV 1.9 and liver SUV 2.8) from 19.9 (re-biopsy) revealed Lugano 3 (which uses the same Deauville scale for NHL).

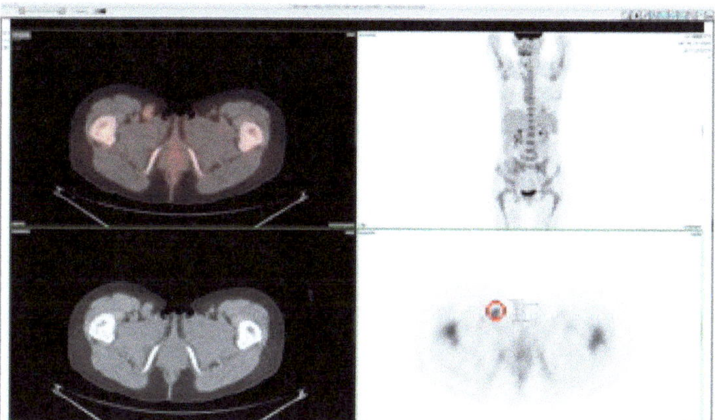

PET after four cycles of R-CHOP showed no uptake. Lugano 1

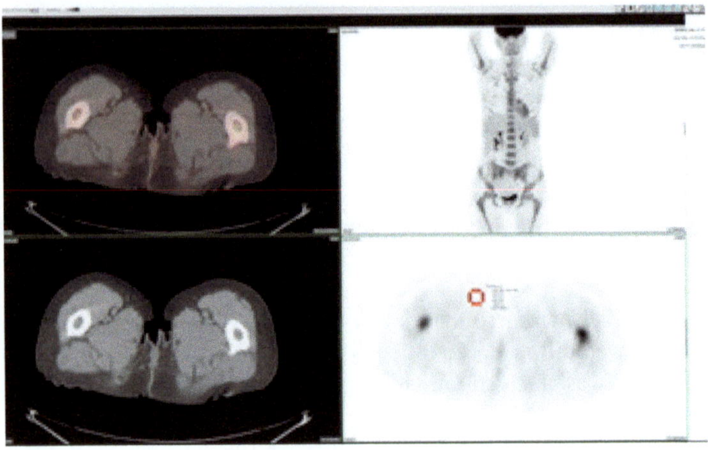

Reference

Wong CYO, Thie J, Parling-Lynch KJ, et al. Investigating the existence of quantum metabolic values in non-Hodgkin's lymphoma by F-18 FDG PET. Mol Imaging Biol. 2007;9(1):43–9.

Chapter 4
Case 4: Metabolic Phenotypes in Different Neoplasms

A: Baseline PET in a known transformed lymphoma at right inguinal node (SUV 19.9) with the maximum SUV at abdomen being 34.1 was consistent with pathological diagnosis of diffuse large B-cell lymphoma (Case 3). (1) What is the tracer? (2) Is a right thyroid uptake (SUV 5.5) a lymphoma or separate adenoma or cancer?

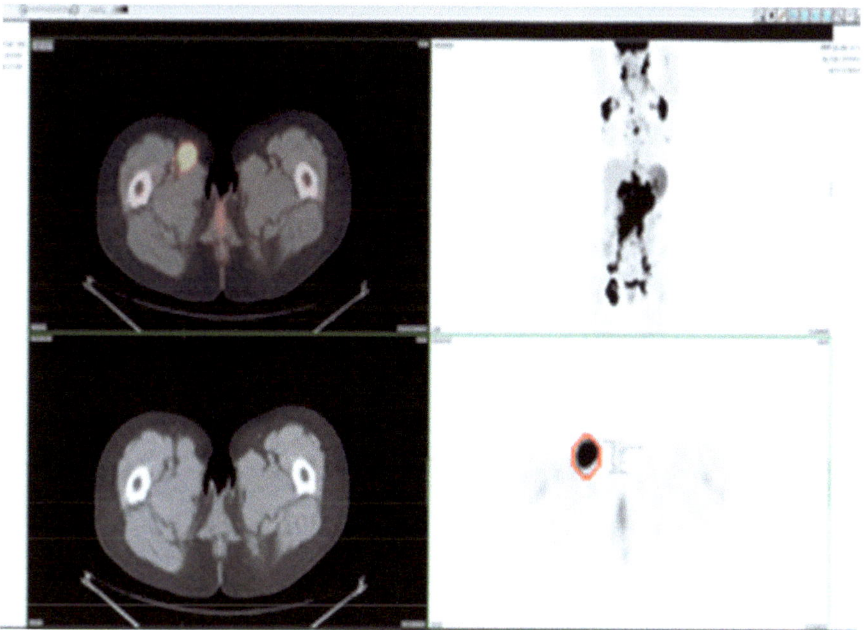

C. Y. O. Wong, D. Wu, *Phenotypic Oncology PET*,
https://doi.org/10.1007/978-3-031-09737-9_4

B: PET after four cycles of R-CHOP showed no uptake except for persistent thyroid uptake (red circle). (1) What is the response? (2) What do you recommend for right thyroid uptake?

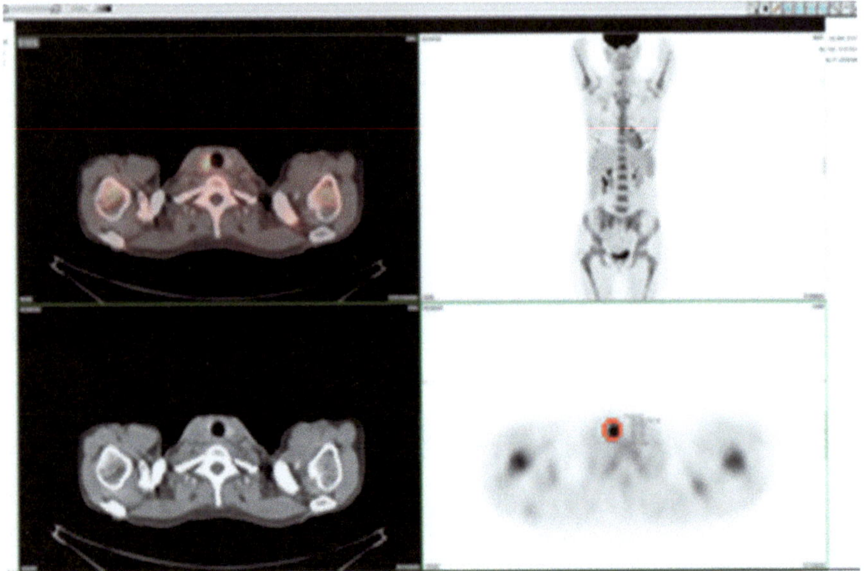

4.1 Case 4: Interpretation and Teaching

A1: F-18 FDG.
A2: No. PET indicated an aggressive lymphoma (DLBCL) inside the abdomen (SUV 34.1). But the thyroid uptake is too low to be compatible of DLBCL uptake. Thus, it is likely a separate adenoma or thyroid cancer.
B1: Lugano 1 complete response.
B2: Ultrasound evaluation. FNA showed papillary thyroid cancer.

Teaching Point 1 Thyroid lymphoma is a rare cancer constituting 1–2% of all thyroid cancers and less than 2% of lymphomas. Thyroid lymphomas are classified as non-Hodgkin's B-cell lymphomas in the majority of cases, although Hodgkin's lymphoma of the thyroid has also been identified.

Teaching Point 2 In general, the higher the metabolic uptake, the more aggressive the tumor. The thyroid nodule usually has a low SUV from adenoma or well-differentiated thyroid. Any focal uptake warrants further evaluation as 10–20% is thyroid cancer like a cold nodule on thyroid scan.

Reference

Sakorafas GH, Kokkoris P, Farley DR. Primary thyroid lymphoma: diagnostic and therapeutic dilemmas. Surg Oncol. 2010;19(4):124–9.

Chapter 5
Case 5: Marrow Involvement in Non-Hodgkin's Lymphoma

A: Baseline PET after two cycles of chemotherapy for NHL. (1) What is the tracer? (2) What is the stage of this lymphoma? (3) How is the aggressiveness of the lymphoma?

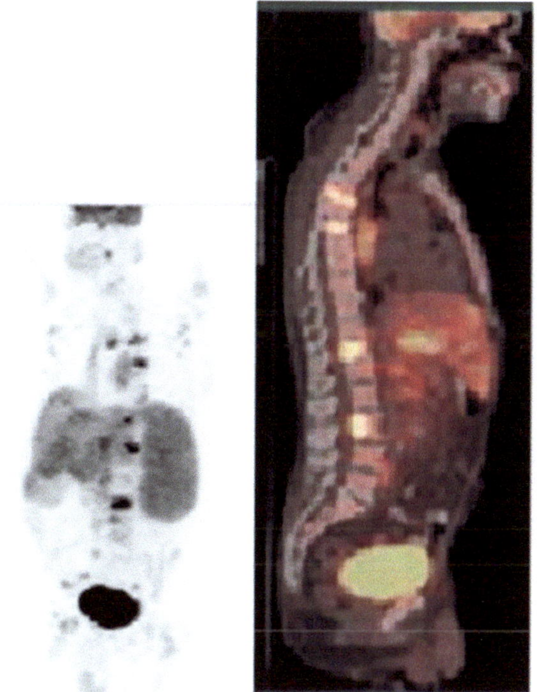

C. Y. O. Wong, D. Wu, *Phenotypic Oncology PET*, https://doi.org/10.1007/978-3-031-09737-9_5

B: The four-cycle posttreatment PET. (1) What is the response? (2) Is there splenic involvement? (3) How is bone marrow response?

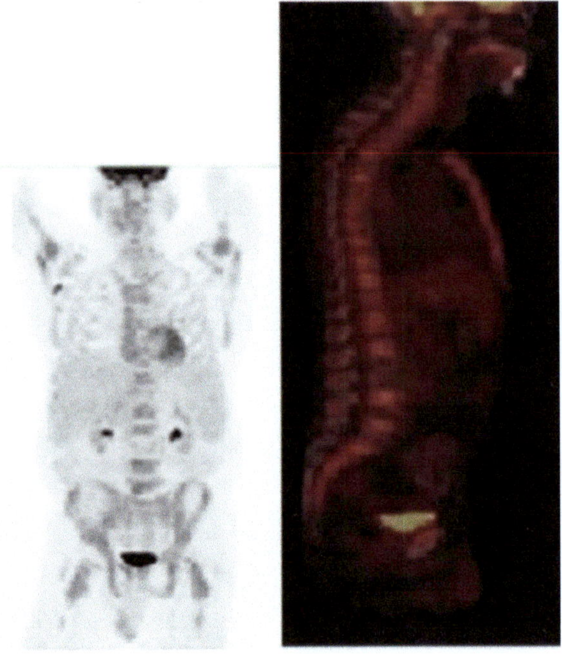

5.1   Case 5: Interpretation and Teaching

A1:   F-18 FDG.

A2:   Stage IV lymphoma.

A3:   Aggressive lymphoma with biopsy showing grade IIIB follicular B-cell lymphoma.

Teaching Point 1 The higher the metabolic uptake, the more aggressive the lymphoma. The PET metabolic phenotype is consistent with high-grade NHL. The focal uptake in marrow renders marrow aspiration unnecessary.

B1:   The patient who received R-CHOP had a complete response. Lugano (Deauville) 1.

B2:   There is bulky splenic involvement by lymphoma which responded well to chemotherapy.

B3:   All the prior areas of focal uptake had decreased uptake showing excellent response or chemosensitivity.

Teaching Point 2 Since some marrow has generalized augmentation in the post-treatment PET, the marrow uptake after treatment is the uninvolved marrow. The baseline focal uptake showed decreased uptake after therapy; this is a retrospective confirmation of marrow involvement. In the case of uniform marrow uptake in baseline PET, any areas of focal decreased marrow uptake after therapy may provide metabolic evidence of potentially undetected marrow disease in these sites.

Reference

Tang BF, Patel MM, Wong RH, et al. Revisiting the marrow metabolic changes after chemotherapy in lymphoma: a step towards personalized care. Int J Mol Imaging. 2011;942063

Chapter 6
Case 6: Hip Pain in Lymphoma

A: Baseline (left) and 3-month posttreatment (right) PET. (1) What is the tracer? (2) Which type of lymphoma? (3) How is the response?

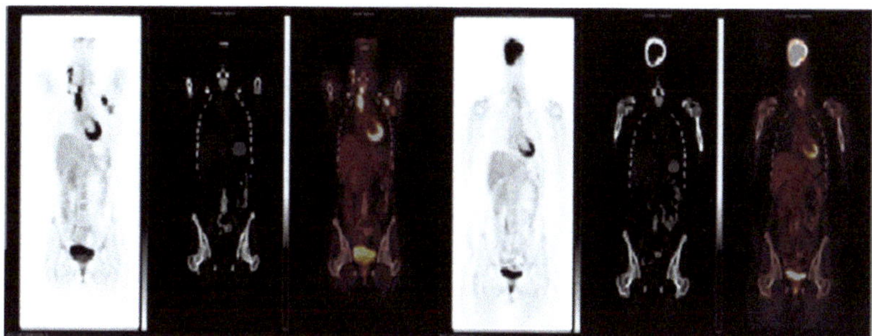

B: Six-month posttreatment PET to evaluate right hip pain. (1) Is there recurrence? (2) What is the cause? (3) How do you confirm the diagnosis?

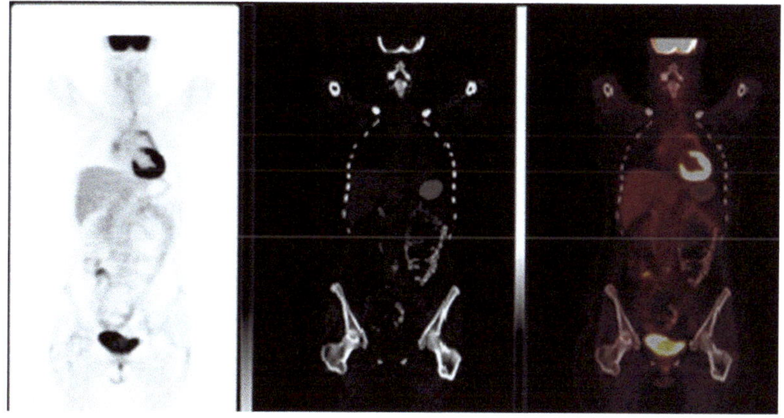

C. Y. O. Wong, D. Wu, *Phenotypic Oncology PET*,
https://doi.org/10.1007/978-3-031-09737-9_6

6.1 Case 6: Interpretation and Teaching

A1:   F-18 FDG.

A2:   High-grade non-Hodgkin's lymphoma.
      Teaching point: Non-Hodgkin's lymphoma. Uptake is much higher than liver
      and even like the intense cardiac uptake is compatible with biopsy showing
      diffuse large B-cell lymphoma.

A3:   The patient who received R-CHOP had a complete response. Lugano 1.

B1:   No recurrence. The mediastinum uptake is from thymic rebound.

B2:   Avascular necrosis from P (prednisone) in R-CHOP with sclerosis at right
      femoral head without FDG uptake.

B3:   MRI hip confirmed PET-CT findings.

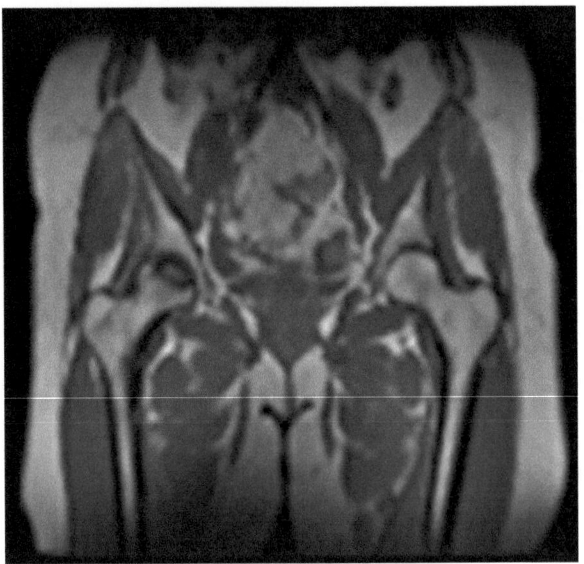

Reference

Thorne JC, Evans WK, Alison RE, et al. Avascular necrosis of bone complicating treatment of
    malignant lymphoma. Am J Med. 1981;71(5):751–8.

Chapter 7
Case 7: Prostate Cancer-Specific PET Agent with Rising PSA

A: PET imaging for PSA 0.2 from 0.15 and < 0.2 ng/ml 1 and 15 years ago. (1) What is the tracer? (2) What is normal distribution (3) How is PET scan starting? (4) What do you see in the prostatectomy bed? (5) What are the interval references? (6) What is the MRI technique to help confirming the diagnosis?

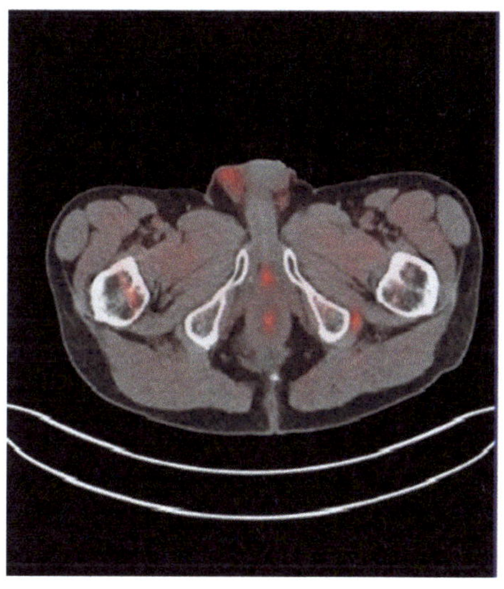 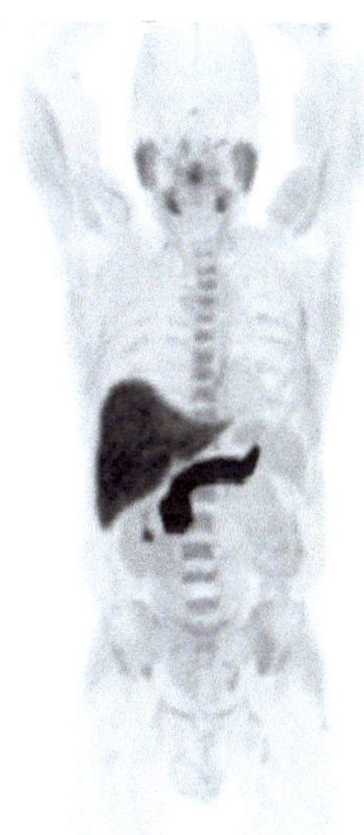

C. Y. O. Wong, D. Wu, *Phenotypic Oncology PET*,
https://doi.org/10.1007/978-3-031-09737-9_7

B: PET images may need to scale down the intensity for evaluation of the pelvic lesions in the whole-body scan. (1) Is the focal update in the left pelvic side wall a nodal recurrence? (2) What is the cause of left pelvic side uptake? (3) How do you confirm the diagnosis?

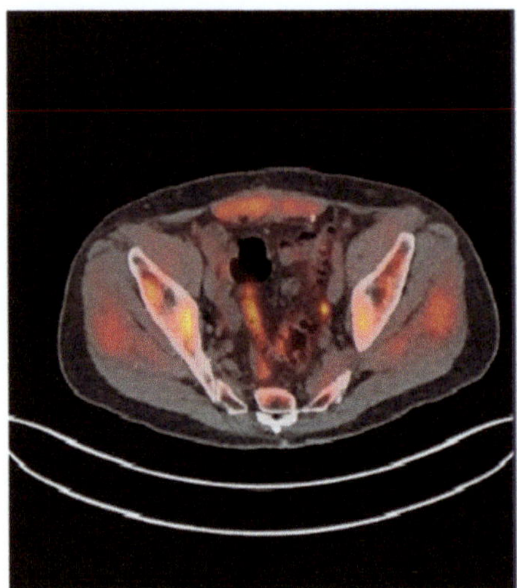 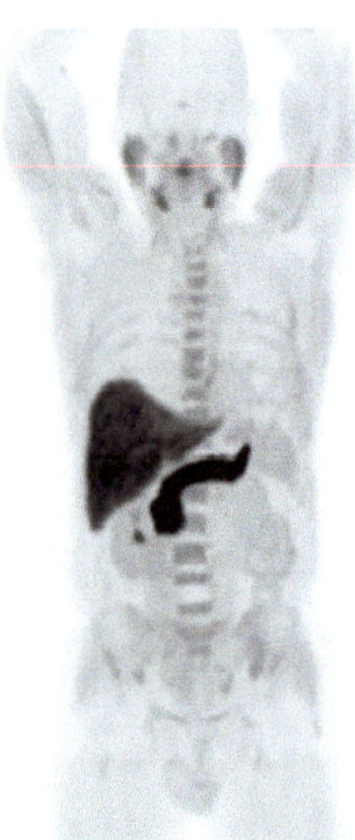

7.1 Case 7: Interpretation and Teaching

A1: F-18 fluciclovine.
A2: High uptake in the liver and pancreas, moderate uptake in the marrow and salivary glands, and low uptake in endocrine glands like pituitary and thyroid are all physiologic.
A3: The PET starts 2.5–3.0 min after injection from the pelvic up to the head.
A4: There is focal uptake in the left side of prostate bed with SUV 2.55.
A5: The internal references are 1.0 cm-diameter blood pool mean SUV 1.28 and 1.5 cm diameter L3 marrow mean SUV 4.28.
A6: Dynamic perfusion subtraction MRI.

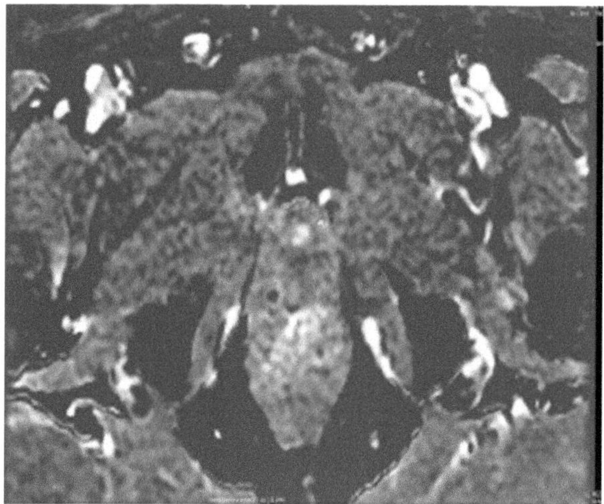

B1: No recurrence in the pelvic nodes.
B2: Distal left ureter tracer retention.
B3: Contrast pelvic MRI.

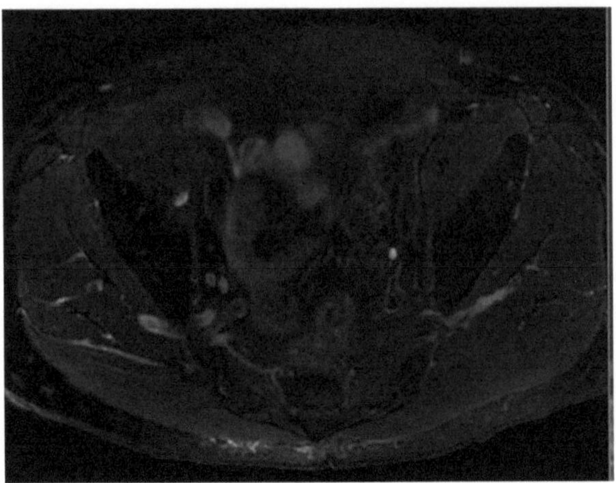

The patient received antiandrogen and radiation and PSA decreased to <0.05 ng/ml.

Reference

Schuster DM, Nanni C, Fanti S, et al. Anti-1-amino-3-18F-Fluorocyclobutane-1-carboxylic acid: physiologic uptake patterns, incidental findings, and variants that may simulate disease. J Nucl Med. 2014;55(12):1986–92.

Chapter 8
Case 8: Brain Tumor Evaluation

A: PET imaging after radiation therapy for glioblastoma multiforme. Uptake ratio of the right lateral temporal lobe to normal tissue is greater than (T/N) 1.4. (1) What is the tracer? (2) Is a seizure focus? (3) What is the diagnosis?

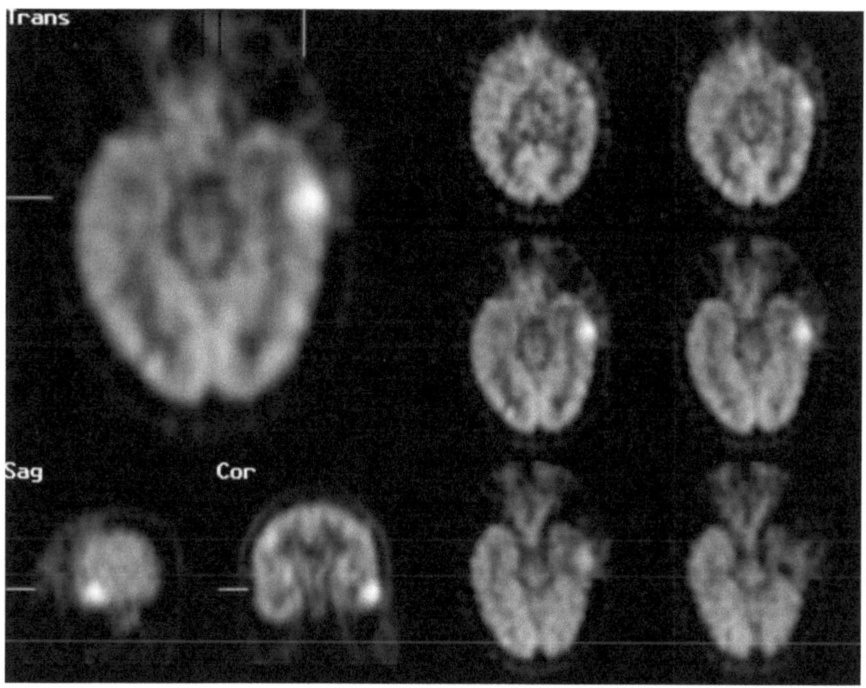

8.1   Case 8: Interpretation and Teaching

A1:   F-18 FDG.
A2:   No. High uptake in right lateral temporal lobe cannot be seizure focus as it does not activate the ipsilateral thalamus and/or cross-activate contralateral cerebellum.
A3:   The T/N ratio is greater than 1.4 suggesting a tumor recurrence.

Teaching Point   Brain evaluation by FDG PET is not only anato-molecular findings but also a functional network connection.

Reference

Wu DF. Clinical nuclear medicine neuroimaging—an instructional casebook. Cham, Switzerland: Springer; 2020.

Chapter 9
Case 9: Metabolic Phenotype in a Slowly Growing Lung Cancer

C. Y. O. Wong, D. Wu, *Phenotypic Oncology PET*

A: Baseline PET showed a small right lung nodule (SUV 0.8) without prior imaging data. (1) What is the tracer? (2) Is the right lung nodule uptake significant?

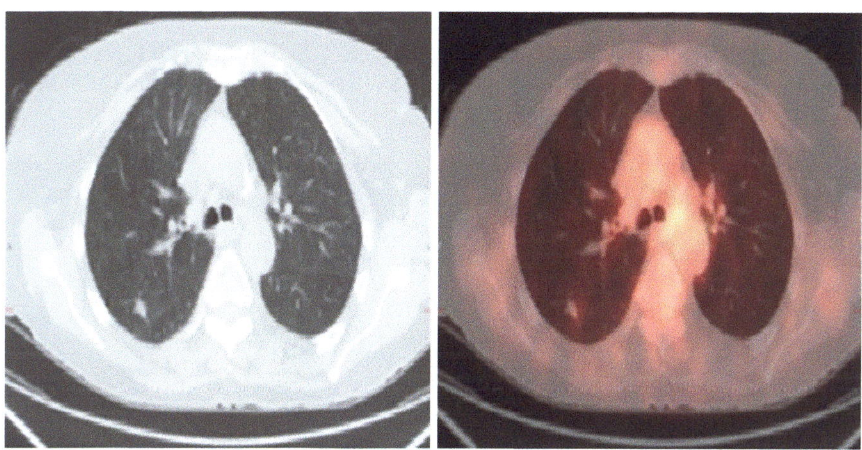

© The Author(s), under exclusive license to Springer Nature
Switzerland AG 2022
C. Y. O. Wong, D. Wu, *Phenotypic Oncology PET*,
https://doi.org/10.1007/978-3-031-09737-9_9

B: Dedicated CT chest 6 months later showed no significant changes in size. Repeated PET-CT showed SUV 2.7 (reference mediastinal blood pool SUV at subcarinal level 2.2). (1) What is the new finding? (2) Is the right lung nodule uptake significant?

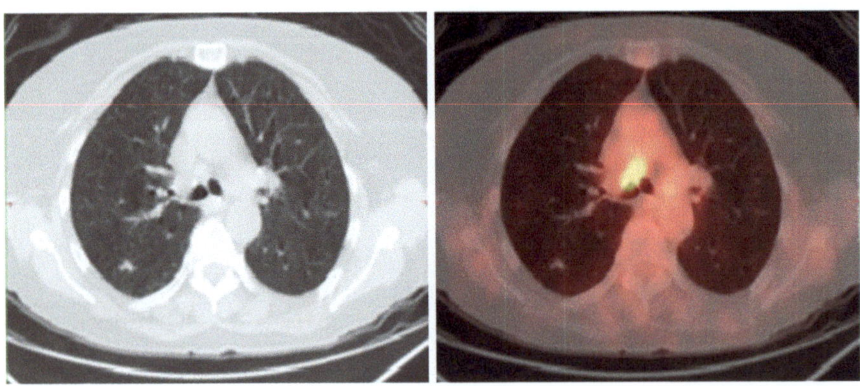

C: Negative mediastinal biopsy after last PET-CT. Repeated PET 1 year later showed SUV 4.7 at the right lung nodule. (1) What is the PET diagnosis? (2) What is likely tumor phenotype?

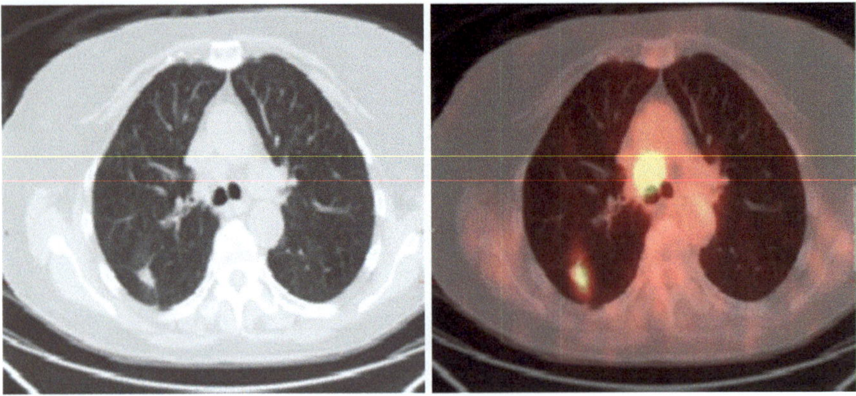

9.1 Case 9: Interpretation and Teaching

A1:   F-18 FDG.
A2:   Yes. PET indicated a focal uptake in the right upper lobe, indicating at least some suspicion of malignancy despite low SUV.

Teaching Point 1 Nonsmoking history does not exclude low-grade cancer let alone there is also secondary smoking. Any growing or new nodule is likely a neoplastic change until proven otherwise. Due to lack of prior imaging, a 3–6 month follow-up PET-CT is likely to be helpful for low metabolic rate tumors such as bronchioalveolar carcinoma (BAC) or low-grade adenocarcinoma.

B1:   Precarinal uptake.
B2:   Yes, despite very low uptake because of new precarinal uptake, suggesting metastasis.

Teaching Point 2 In general, the newly diagnosed primary lung cancer has higher metabolic uptake than the nodal metastasis except for the well-differentiated adenocarcinoma or BAC. Unfortunately, mediastinal biopsy was negative.

C1:   Primary lung cancer with mediastinal nodal metastasis. Stage IIIA.
C2:   Low-grade adenocarcinoma. It is confirmed by repeated mediastinal biopsy.

Reference

Wang Y, Ma S, Dong M, et al. Evaluation of the factors affecting the maximum standardized uptake value of metastatic lymph nodes in different histological types of non-small cell lung cancer on PET-CT. BMC Pulm Med. 2015;15:20.

Chapter 10
Case 10: Metabolic Phenotype in Lung Metastasis from Colon Cancer

A: Baseline PET metastatic colon cancer to liver (left) and post-segmentectomy PET (right). (1) What is the tracer? (2) Is PET negative after liver surgery?

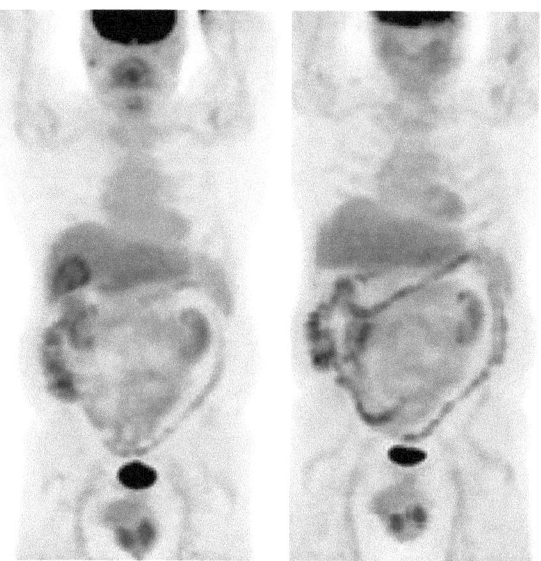

C. Y. O. Wong, D. Wu, *Phenotypic Oncology PET*, https://doi.org/10.1007/978-3-031-09737-9_10

B: Baseline PET-CT.(1) Are there lung nodules?

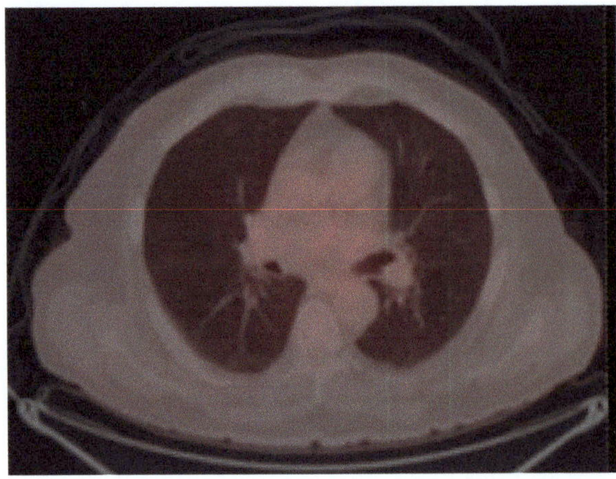

C: PET-CT after 6 months of segmentectomy. (1) Are there lung nodules? (2) What is the diagnosis?

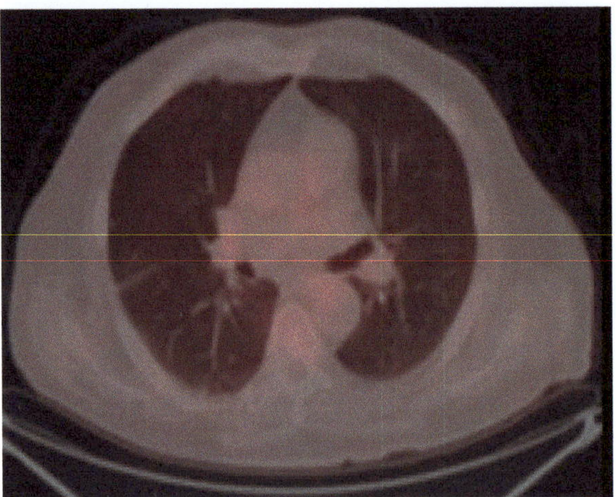

10.1 Case 10: Interpretation and Teaching

A1: F-18 FDG.
A2: Yes. PET is negative for avid tumor foci.

Teaching Point 1 Non-avid metastases do occur. Any growing or new lesions are likely metastasis until proven otherwise. In colon cancers, mucinous type may not have FDG uptake.

B1: No.
C1: Yes. Multiple small right lung nodules appear, and none is avid.

Teaching Point 2 In general, the new lung nodules are assumed to be metastasis irrespective of FDG avidity.

C2: Low-grade metastatic adenocarcinoma from colon cancer.

Reference

Berger KL, Nicholson SA, Dehdashti F, et al. FDG PET evaluation of mucinous neoplasms correlation of FDG uptake with histopathologic features. Am J Roentgenol. 2000;174:1005–8.

Chapter 11
Case 11: PET and Bone Scans in Non-Small Cell Lung Cancer

A: Baseline PET (right) and bone (left) scans in a 52-year-old nonsmoker with adenocarcinoma of the lung. (1) What are the tracers for PET and bone scans? (2) What is the likelihood of EGFR positivity? (3) What is the stage of lung cancer?

C. Y. O. Wong, D. Wu, *Phenotypic Oncology PET*,
https://doi.org/10.1007/978-3-031-09737-9_11

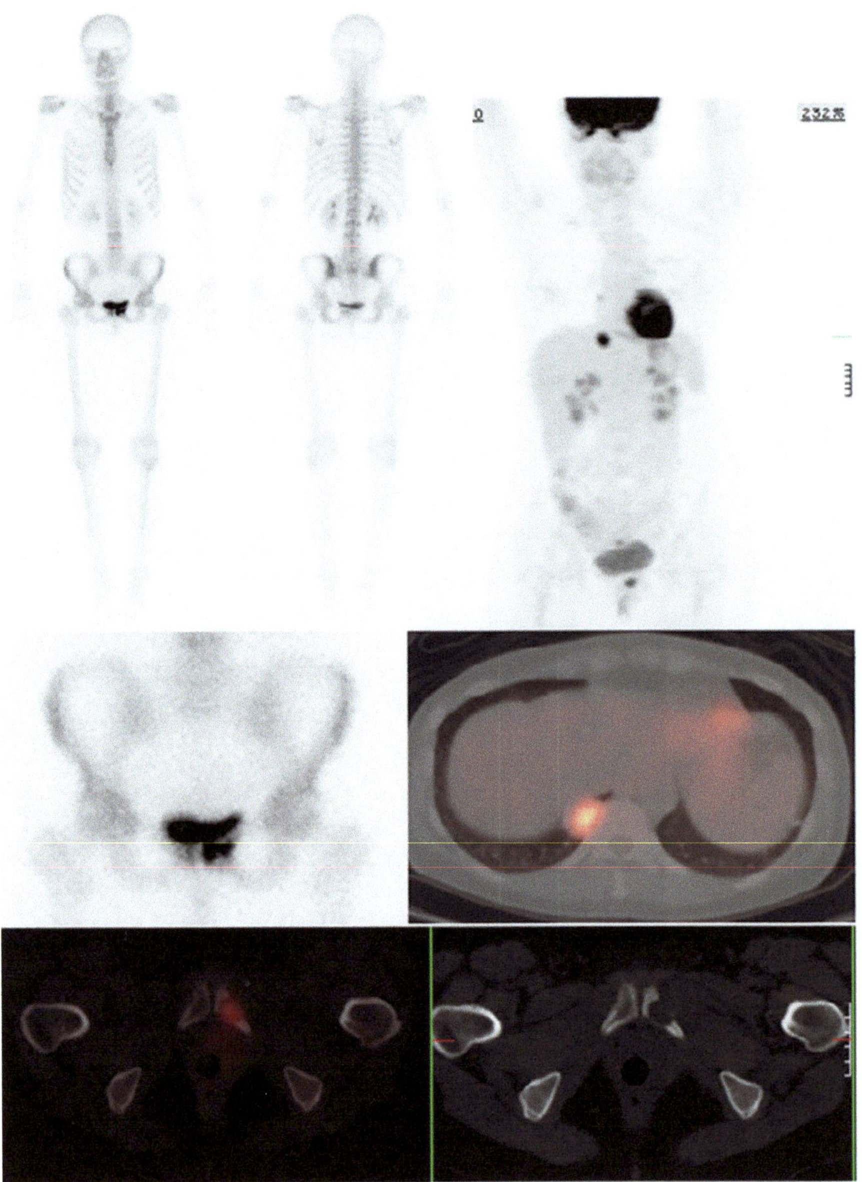

B: Follow-up PET (middle row and upper left) and bone (lower row and upper right) scan after Tacerva. (1) What is the response in primary cancer? (2) What is the response in bone metastasis? What will be the next step?

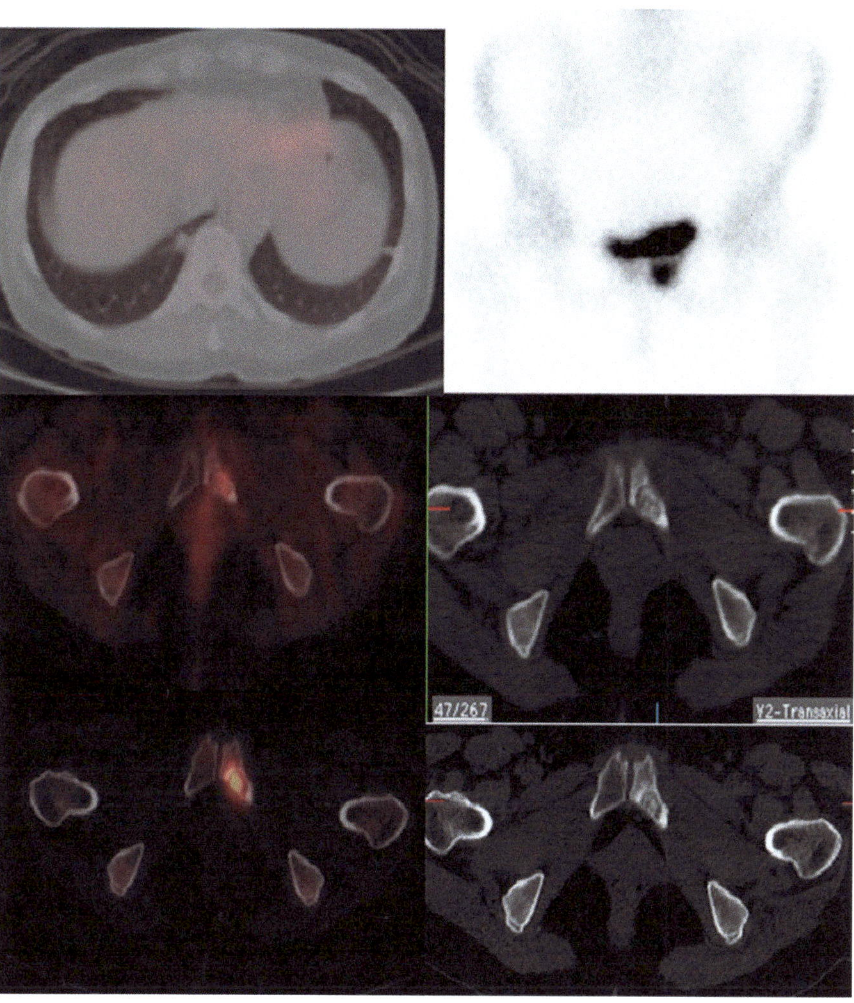

11.1   Case 11: Interpretation and Teaching

A1:   F-18 FDG and Tc-99m MDP.
A2:   There is a high chance of positive EGFR by history and low metabolic phenotype.
A3:   Stage IV.

Teaching Point 1 Besides being a nonsmoker female with adenocarcinoma, the lower the metabolic uptake, the higher chance for EGFR positive which is confirmed by FISH.

B1:   Excellent response to targeted therapy.
B2:   Partial response in left pubic bone with residual mild uptake and sclerotic changes from original lytic lesion in CT, suggesting partial healing process. Localized SBRT will be the logical approach.

Teaching Point 2 Healing starts with decreased FDG uptake and bone sclerosis. But complete healing requires negative bone uptake.

PET after radiation showed negative uptake in left pubic bone with more sclerosis:

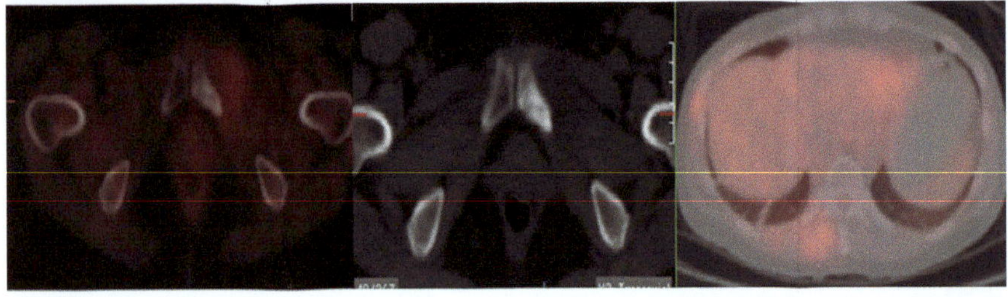

Teaching Point 3 Complete healing in this bone is important to prevent fracture and limping gait.

Reference

Takamochi K, Mogushi K, Kawaji H, et al. Correlation of EGFR or KRAS mutation status with 18F-FDG uptake on PET-CT scan in lung adenocarcinoma. PLoS One. 2017;12(4):e0175622.

Chapter 12
Case 12: Neuroendocrine Cancer of the Ileum

A: Initial PET imaging for restaging breast cancer (1) What is the tracer? (2) What is the finding on MIP?

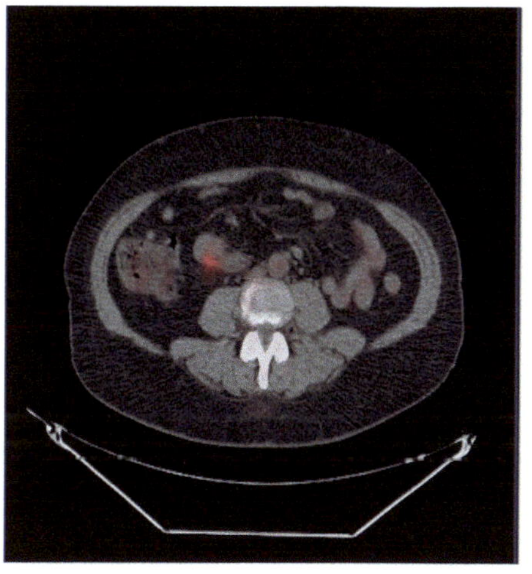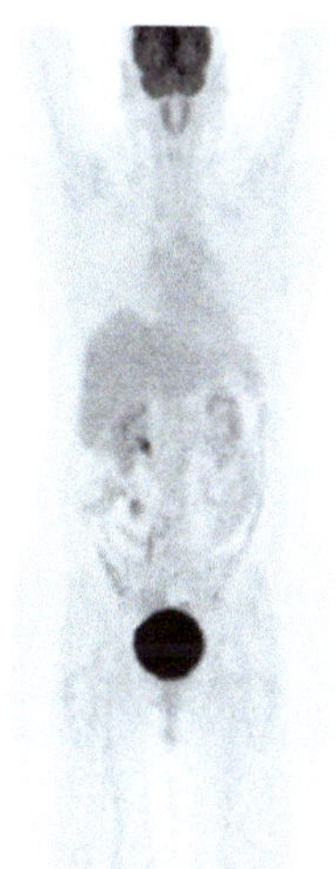

C. Y. O. Wong, D. Wu, *Phenotypic Oncology PET*,
https://doi.org/10.1007/978-3-031-09737-9_12

B: Another type of PET imaging. (1) What is the tracer? (2) What is normal distribution? (3) How is PET scan starting?

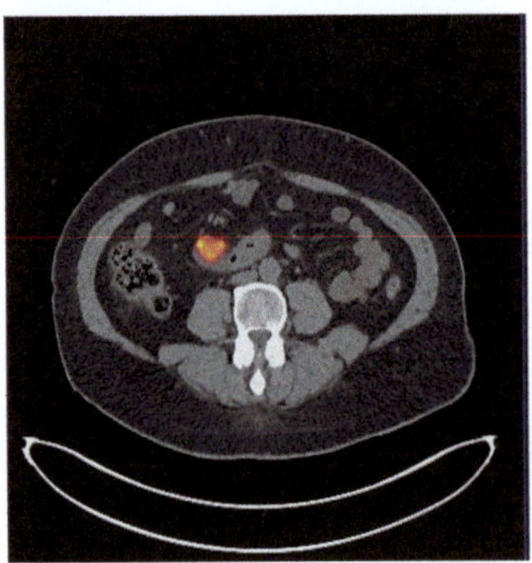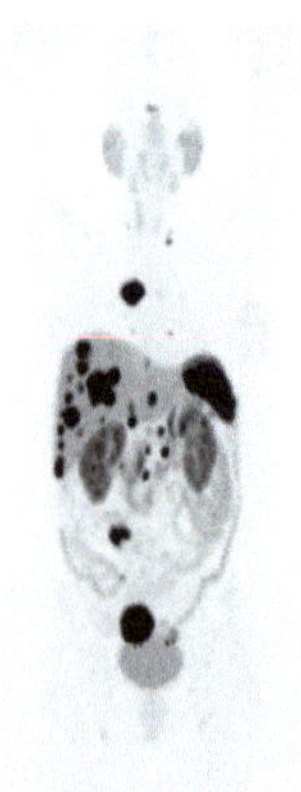

C: PET imaging over pelvis using the tracers in (**a**) left vs. (**b**) right. (1) What is the diagnosis? (2) What is the tumor marker?

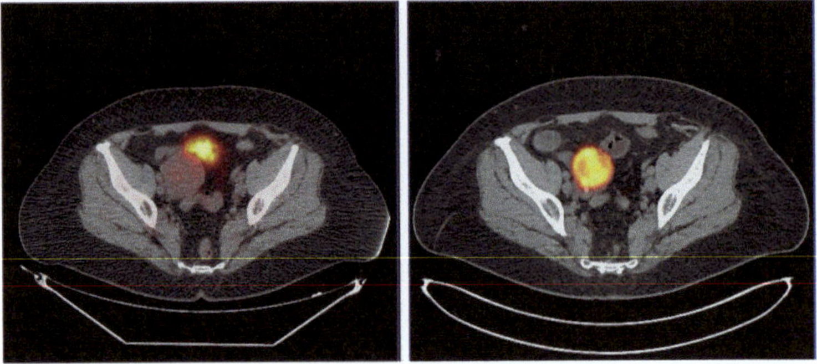

D: PET after surgery and chemotherapy on monthly octreotide with serum chromogranin A 139 ng/ml. (1) What are the major findings? (2) What is the overall tumor load?

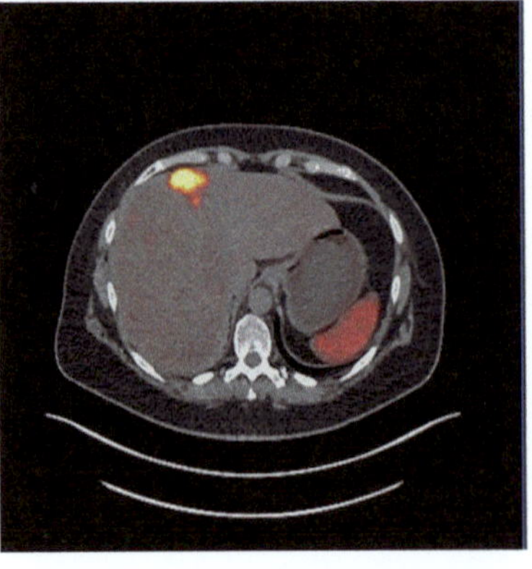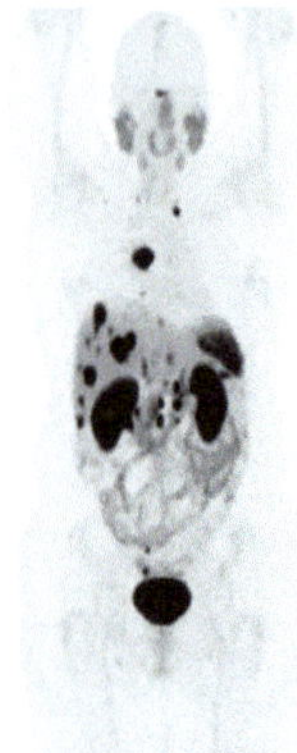

12.1 Case 12: Interpretation and Teaching

A1:   F-18 FDG.
A2:   No recurrent breast cancer with nonspecific terminal ileal uptake.

B1:   Ga-68 DOTA-DPhen1.
B2:   High uptake in the spleen, moderate uptake in the pituitary and liver, and low uptake in the thyroid, adrenal, salivary glands, and pancreas are all physiologic. Normal renal excretion.
B3:   The PET starts about 60 min after injection from the head to pelvis.

C1:   Neuroendocrine tumor.

Teaching Point 1 Well-differentiated tumor has low FDG uptake but high DOTA uptake, another reflection of tumor phenotype.

C2:   Serum chromogranin A which was at 191 ng/ml (well-differentiated tumor, G2) after surgical resection of terminal ileum and BSO showing bilateral ovarian metastasis.

D1:   Diffuse metastases to the liver. Others are right mid thoracic paraspinal and scattered metastases in the left lower anterior cervical/thoracic inlet, retroperitoneum, and right posterior pelvis.
D2:   No significant changes in overall tumor metastatic load are noted.

E: PET images after liver-directed therapy with doxorubicin bead chemoembolization showing minor local response with chromogranin A at 110 ng/ml.

Teaching Point 2 Liver tumor load assessment is important in liver-directed therapy including Y-90 microspheres.

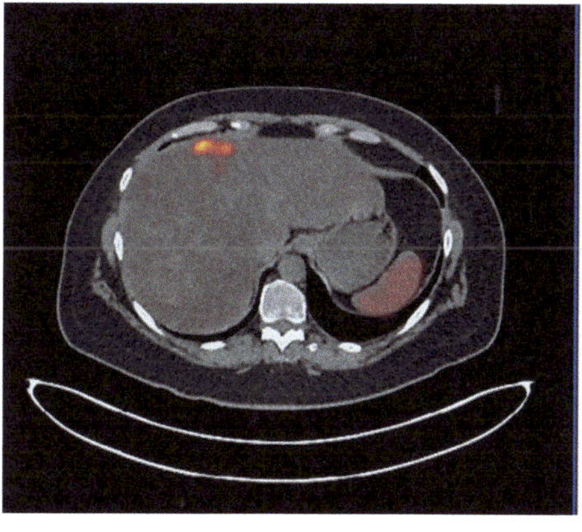
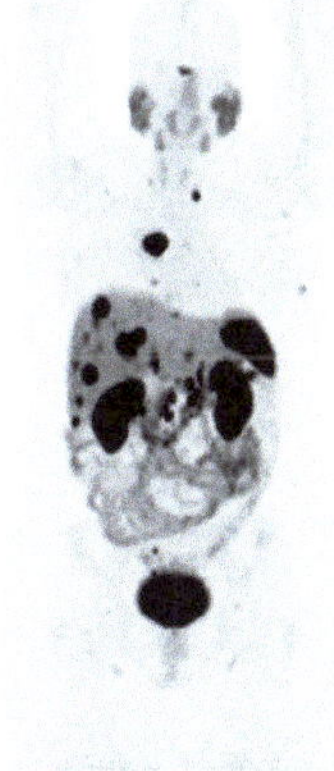

Reference

Kuyumcu S, Özkan ZG, et al. Physiological and tumoral uptake of 68Ga-DOTATATE: standardized uptake values and challenges in interpretation. Ann Nucl Med. 2013;27:538–45.

Chapter 13
Case 13: Coexisting Different PET Tumor Phenotypes

A: Low-grade follicular lymphoma 5 years ago with marrow involvement and carcinoid tumor at ileal region and metastases to the lung, liver, ovaries, and nodes 4 years ago status post-multiple surgical resection and lymphadenectomy and on octreotide every 3 weeks. PET showed SUV at 12 mm right cervical node (left panel 7.41 and right panel 8.17). (1) What are the tracers? (2) What are the findings on MIP? (3) What is most likely phenotype for the right cervical node?

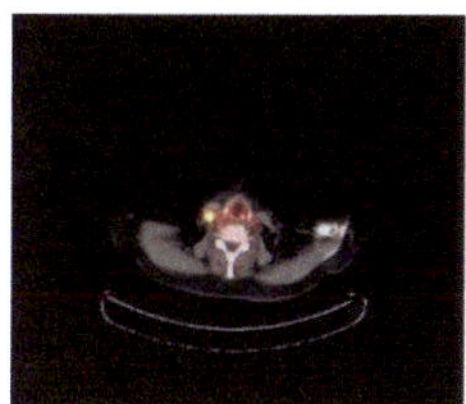 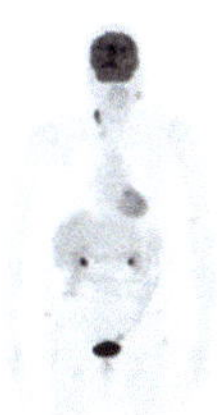 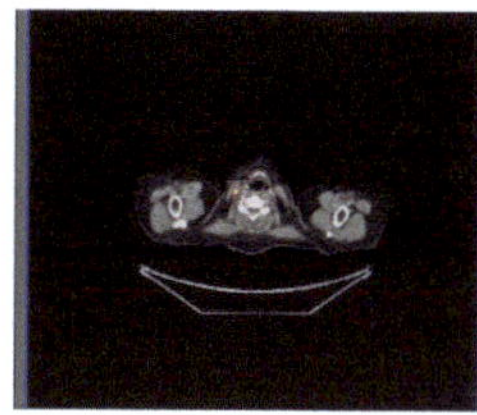 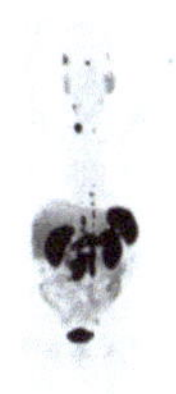

B: Chest section on PET imaging (17 × 13 mm lung nodule SUV, left panel 2.31 and right panel 35.69, and 1 cm right retrocrural node SUV, left panel 1.28 and right panel 19.68). (1) What is tumor phenotype in lung nodule? (2) What is tumor phenotype in retrocrural node?

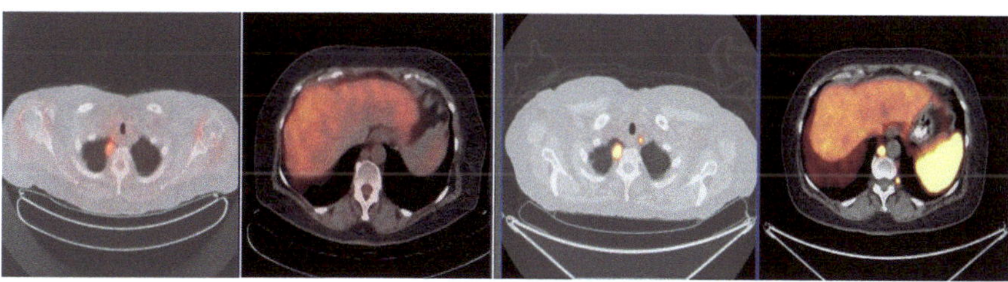

C. Y. O. Wong, D. Wu, *Phenotypic Oncology PET*,
https://doi.org/10.1007/978-3-031-09737-9_13

C: Abdomen and pelvis on PET imaging. There is a large conglomerate of nodes in the retroperitoneum and mesentery (SUV left 1.37 and 1.93 and right panel 35.38 and 16.28). (1) What is (are) tumor phenotype(s) of the nodes in the retroperitoneum and mesentery?

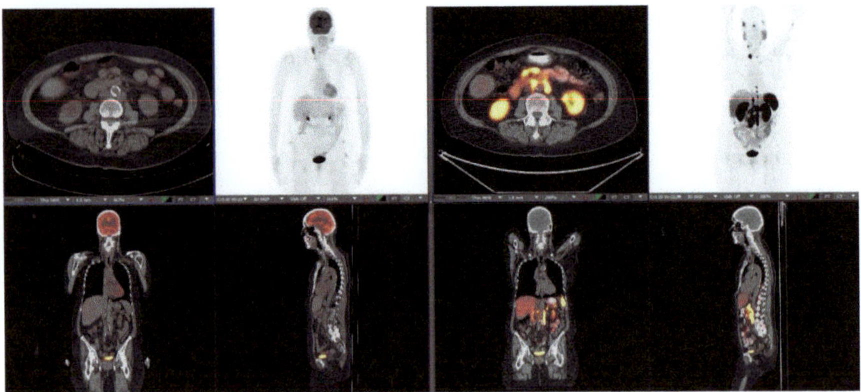

13.1   Case 13: Interpretation and Teaching

A1:   F-18 FDG (13.3 mCi) and Ga-68 DOTA-DPhen1 (DOTATATE, 5.9 mCi).

A2:   Different patterns of uptake for these tracers, both physiologically and pathologically.

A3:   Right cervical node is likely from follicular lymphoma which is confirmed by biopsy to be grade 3A with CD20/21+ and MIB-1 being 10–20%.

Reference SUV FDG (cf=compared to DOTATATE):

1. The mediastinal blood pool 2.09 (cf 1.48)
2. The right lobe of the liver 2.89 (cf 4.83)
3. The spleen 1.98 (cf 16.70)
4. The L3 marrow 1.53 (cf 2.38)
5. The right cerebellum 7.92 (cf 0.81)

B1, B2, and C1:   Right lung, left pleura, left high retrotracheal, bilateral para-aortic/retrocrural, retroperitoneal nodes, and mesenteric masses are metastatic neuroendocrine tumors due to high uptake in DOTATATE PET.

Teaching Point 1 Well-differentiated neuroendocrine tumor has low FDG uptake but high DOTATATE uptake, another reflection of tumor phenotype. Serum chromogranin A at 256 ng/ml 2 months ago (normal < 311 ng/ml). Lymphoma is usually low in DOTATATE uptake. The cervical node has low FDG and DOTATATE uptake and thus it is likely follicular lymphoma.

D: Neck PET images another possible tumor phenotype in the left parotid gland measuring 1.2 cm with SUV 4.95 on FDG and 5.51 on DOTATATE.

Teaching Point 2 Warthin's or other benign parotid tumors are quite common incidental findings which may be followed up by ultrasound and/or tissue correlation. Parotid gland tumors account for 80% of all salivary gland neoplasms; 20% of these are malignant, but in daily clinical practice, most parotid masses are operated on before obtaining the final histological diagnosis. FDG avidity can be observed in benign tumors.

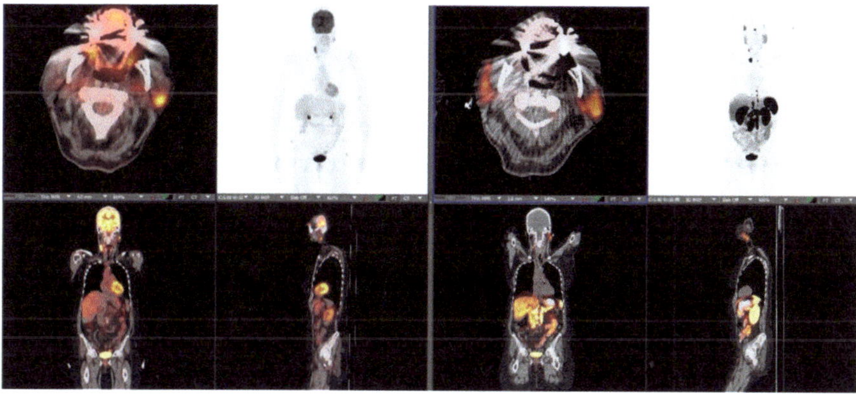

Reference

Ruuska T, Escalante YR, Vaittinen S, et al. Somatostatin receptor expression in lymphomas: a source of false diagnosis of neuroendocrine tumor at Ga-68 DOTANOC PET/CT imaging. Acta Oncologica. 2017;57(2):283–9.

Chapter 14
Case 14: COVID-19 Vaccination and Lung Nodules

A: 54 years year old with smoking history having new right mid lung pulmonary nodule for diagnostic evaluation of lung cancer. COVID-19 vaccination with first dose 25 days and second dose 4 days before PET at the left side with Pfizer vaccine. (1) What is the tracer? (2) What is the likely cause of left axillary lymphadenopathy? (3) What is the next step for avid lung nodules? (4) What is pulmonary function?

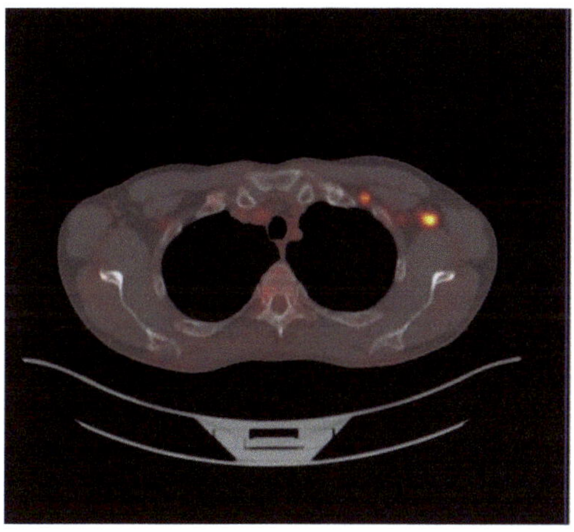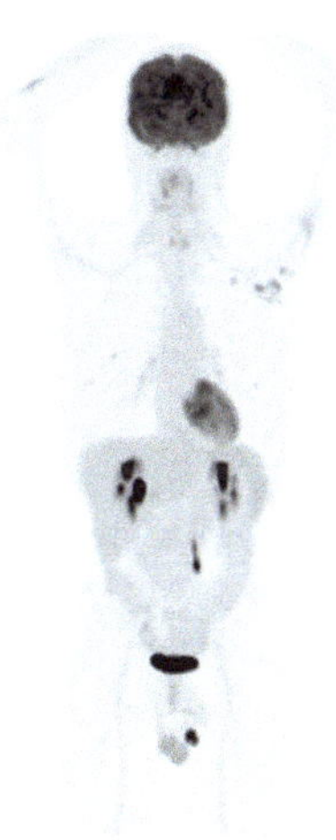

C. Y. O. Wong, D. Wu, *Phenotypic Oncology PET*,
https://doi.org/10.1007/978-3-031-09737-9_14

B: Lung nodules progressed on PET 4 months later. (1) What happens to the left axillary lymphadenopathy? (2) What is the significance of left pleural uptake? (3) What is the next investigation?

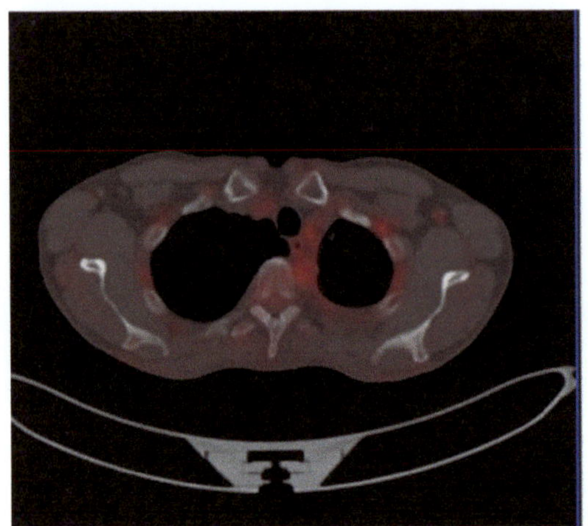 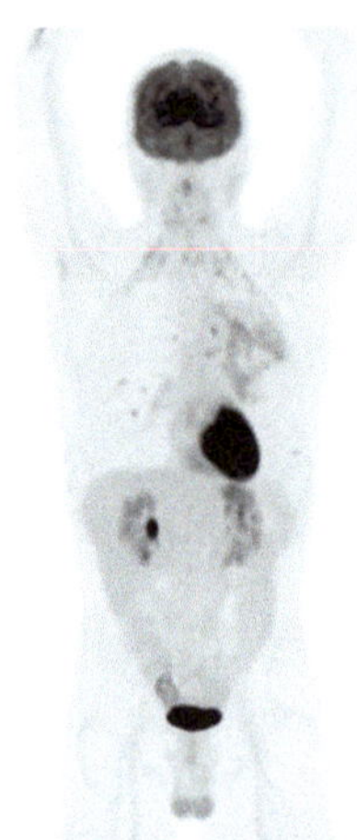

14.1 Case 14: Interpretation and Teaching

A1: F-18 FDG.
A2: Since there is no avid focus on the left chest, the left axillary lymphadenopathy is likely from recent COVID-19 vaccination.
A3: There is avidity on the new (by recent CT to CT comparisons qv infra in D) 1.9 cm likely spiculated pulmonary nodule in the right mid lung together with other new-looking avid nodules (by recent CT to PET-CT comparisons with limitation on different techniques). There is avid bilateral hilar adenopathy. Although these are concerning for possible malignancy, infectious or inflammatory disease is possible in view of relatively short interval appearance of some avid nodules. Suggest short-term imaging follow-up after a trial course of antibiotics in 2–3 weeks.
A4: The use of accessory respiratory and intercostal muscles suggests laborious breathing due to poor pulmonary function from COPD.

C: Biopsies were not to be attempted due to risks associated with severe emphysema. Follow-up PET was ordered.

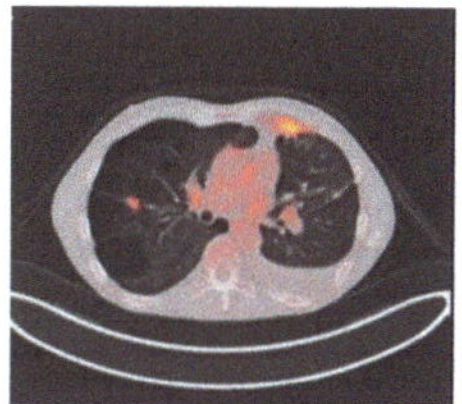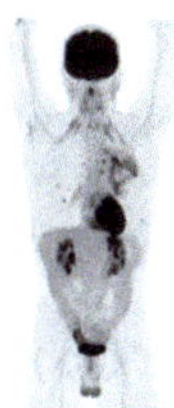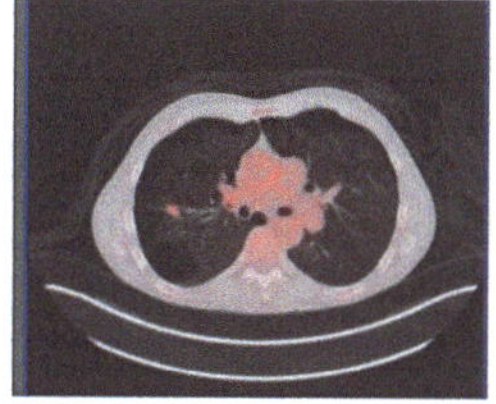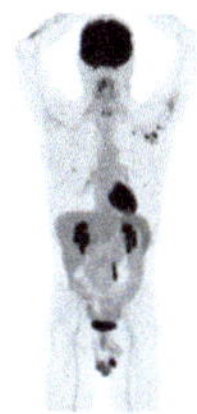

Right mid lung nodule has SUV 4.44 with similar morphology to the last PET SUV 3.14. Mediastinal blood pool has SUV 2.32 from 1.99 on last PET. This together with new or progressing avid nodules is suspicious of metastatic disease.

B1: Resolved.

Teaching Point 1 Inflammation due to recent COVID-19 can last 4–6 weeks. Small-sized and benign-looking nodes with relevant history are the key to correct diagnosis. PET scan is done whenever there is an oncologic indication as 2/3 of cancer will show metabolic progression in 4–6 weeks.

B2: The pleural uptake is suggestive of malignant pleural effusion.
B3: Pleural tap will be next investigation. It was attempted under ultrasound guidance, but the volume was too small to get the fluid.

D: Two CT images 19 months apart with most recent CT (on the left with IV contrast) about 1 month before the first PET showed new right mild lung spiculated nodule with progression of COPD.

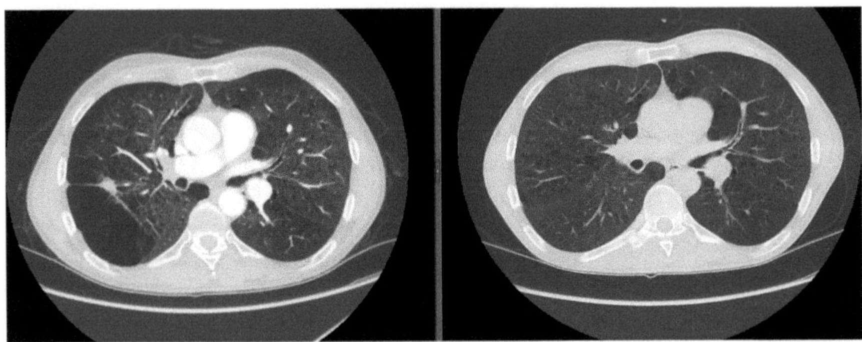

Teaching Point 2 Any new or growing lung nodule irrespective of FDG avidity is suspicious of malignancy. The mild FDG uptake and multicentric foci suggest likely adenocarcinoma.

Reference

McIntosh LJ, Bankier AA, Vijayaraghavan GR, et al. COVID-19 vaccination-related uptake on FDG PET/CT: an emerging dilemma and suggestions for management. AJR. 2021;217:975–83.

Chapter 15
Case 15: COVID-19 Vaccination and Tumor Phenotypes

A: Colon cancer status post-surgery 12 years ago, malignant melanoma of back status post-surgery 11 years ago, right breast cancer status post-right modified radical mastectomy, and chemotherapy 2 years ago. COVID-19 vaccination with first dose 25 days and second dose 4 days before PET at the left side with Pfizer vaccine. (1) What is the tracer? (2) What is the likely cause of left axillary lymphadenopathy? (3)Where is (are) the primary cancer(s)?

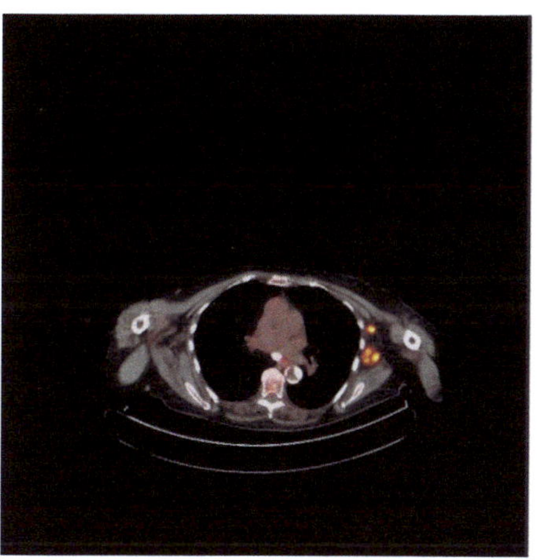 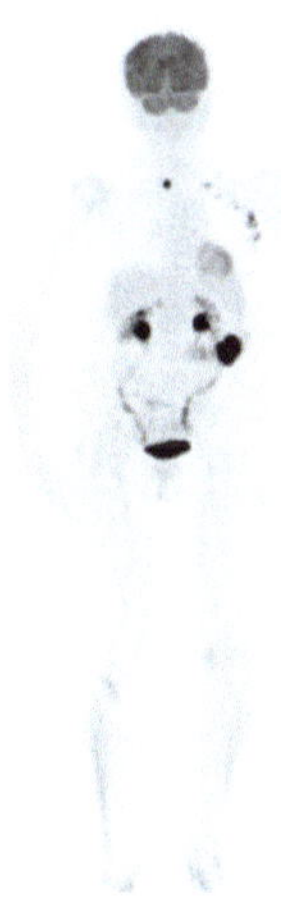

C. Y. O. Wong, D. Wu, *Phenotypic Oncology PET*, https://doi.org/10.1007/978-3-031-09737-9_15

B: Recurrent metastatic colon cancer at splenic flexure with repeated surgery (left hemicolectomy, stage III) 2 months later. Restaging PET was ordered 3 months after the first PET. (1) What happens to the left axillary lymphadenopathy? (2) Does it change in right thyroid uptake? (3) Is there any significant changes in the right adrenal uptake? What is the next investigation?

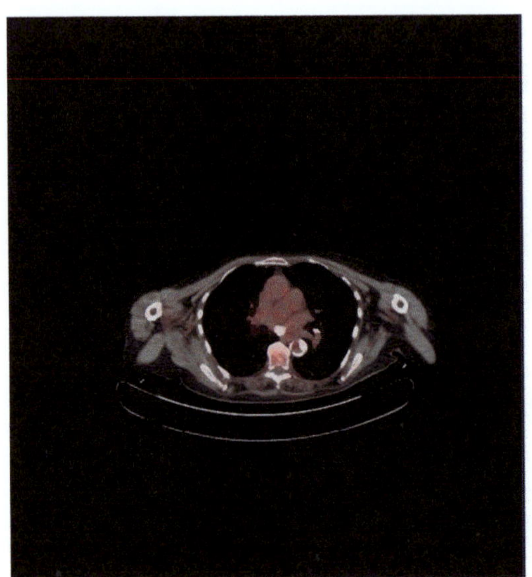
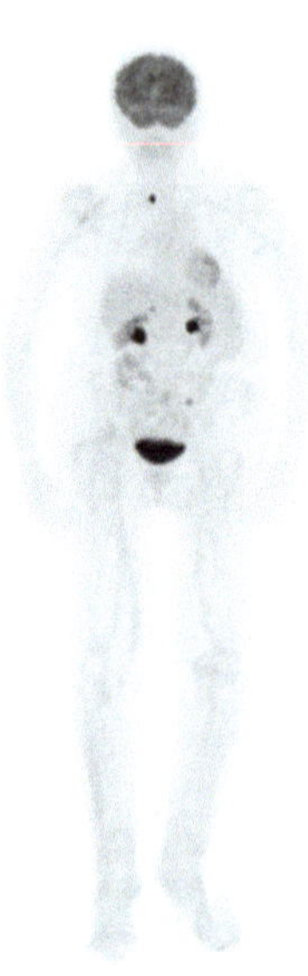

15.1 Case 15: Interpretation and Teaching

A1: F-18 FDG.

A2: Since there is no avid focus on the left breast, the left axillary lymphadenopathy is likely from recent COVID-19 vaccination with deltoid inflammation. Extensive left axillary FDG-avid lymphadenopathy and supraclavicular lymphadenopathy have SUV 8.9 and sizes measuring in supraclavicular node 15 × 9 mm, subpectoral node 9 × 6 mm, and level 1 axillary node 12 × 6 mm. As this case was done in the beginning of vaccination program, left axillary lymph node fine needle aspiration was done showing moderate amount of lymphoid tissue and negative for carcinoma.

A3: Right avid 10 × 8 mm low-attenuation thyroid nodule is detected with SUV 16.2 which is suspicious of new malignancy. Fine needle aspiration was done under ultrasound guidance 1 month later, suspicious for follicular neoplasm (Bethesda category 4), and followed up with endocrinologist. Recurrent metastatic colon cancer at splenic flexure was detected during repeated surgery 2 months later (left hemicolectomy, stage III). Slight nodularity of right adrenal gland has SUV 5.3 suspicious of metastatic disease.

B1: Inflammation due to recent COVID-19 has resolved.

Teaching Point 1 Inflammation due to recent COVID-19 can last 4–6 weeks. Small-sized and benign-looking nodes with relevant history are the key to correct diagnosis.

B2: The 10 × 8 mm low-attenuation nodule right lobe thyroid is again seen with SUV 10.30 which is significantly decreased from prior 16.2 which can be seen in the known thyroid neoplasm with varying TSH (0.70 compared to (cf) 2.02; normal 0.34–4.82 uIU/mL) even without any thyroid medications.

B3: Slight nodularity of right adrenal gland with activity (SUV 4.97 cf 5.3) is higher than the adjacent liver, and thus it is still suspicious of metastatic disease (versus adenoma). Next investigation is MRI or dedicated contrast adrenal CT.

Reference SUV (*cf* = compared to last PET): mediastinal blood pool SUV 1.64 cf 1.20; liver dome SUV 2.30 cf 2.18.

C: Two adrenal PET images showed adrenal uptake, but MRI did reveal any right adrenal nodularity.

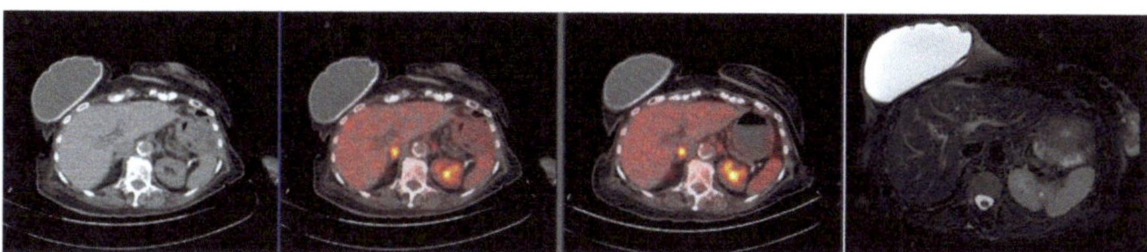

Teaching Point 2 FDG avidity in adrenal gland higher than the liver can rarely be observed in benign adenoma (at about 3%). The hyperplasia is usually bilateral. Follow-up imaging is required for further investigation if the activity is significantly higher than the liver.

Reference

Dong A, Cui Y, Wang Y, et al. F18-FDG PET/CT of adrenal lesions. AJR. 2014;203:245–52.

Chapter 16
Case 16: Breast and Ovarian Uptake

A: Restaging PET-CT for a 42-year-old female with adenocarcinoma of sigmoid colon with biopsy confirmed hepatic metastatic involvement, treated with surgical resection, chemotherapy, and Avastin. There is avidity over the left dense breast SUV 2.08 (prior PET 1.16) and right dense breast SUV 1.82 (prior PET 1.39) without changes in configuration. Reference mediastinal blood pool activity SUV 1.88 (prior 1.44). (1) What is the tracer? (2) Is breast and ovarian uptake pathological or physiologic? (3) What is PET impression?

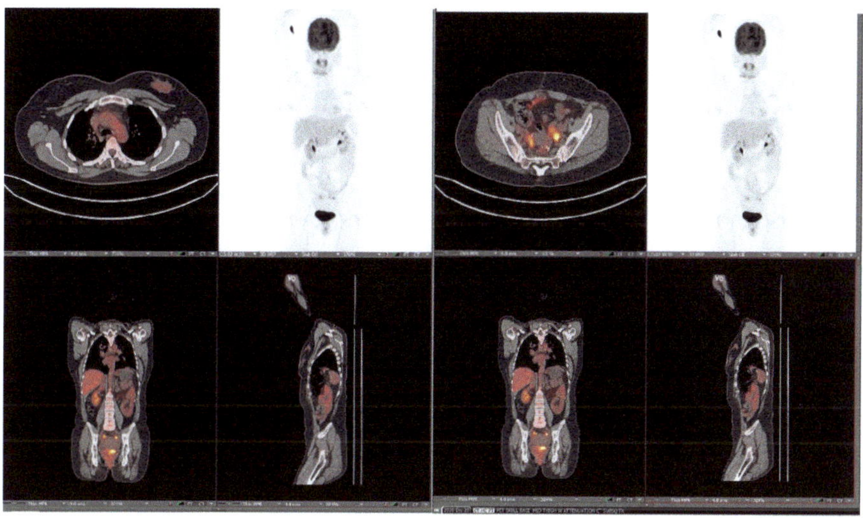

C. Y. O. Wong, D. Wu, *Phenotypic Oncology PET*,
https://doi.org/10.1007/978-3-031-09737-9_16

B: Recent bilateral mammogram *with tomosynthesis and* another restaging PET 31 months ago. (1) What is the PET diagnosis? (2) Is there ovarian uptake?

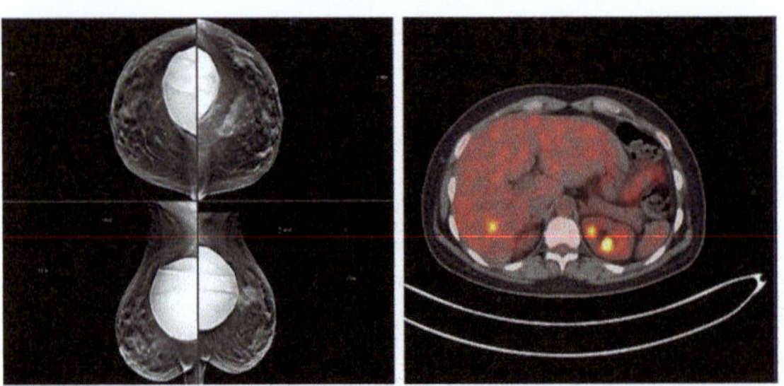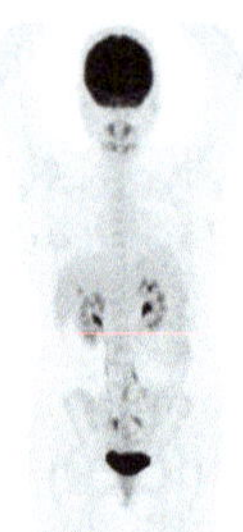

16.1   Case 16: Interpretation and Teaching

A1:   F-18 FDG.

A2:   There is increasing avidity over the left dense breast, and right dense breast without changes in configuration is likely physiologic when the progesterone level is high. The bilateral ovarian uptake which parallels the breast uptake is also physiologic.

A3:   No evidence of FDG-avid residual/recurrent malignancy, with potential limitation on small non-avid foci on the liver. Suggest correlation with CEA and/or PET.

Teaching Point Avidity over dense breast tissue may be related to the menstrual cycle (progesterone) as seen in the ovarian uptake in current PET scan. Correlation with mammogram is suggested as indicated.

B1:   There is a focus of increased uptake (SUV 5.28) in the posterior right lobe of the liver suggesting metastasis.

B2:   The bilateral ovarian uptake which parallels the breast uptake is also physiologic. Recent mammogram is negative.

C: The prior PET was done 7 months ago in low progesterone level status where there is no uptake in the breasts.

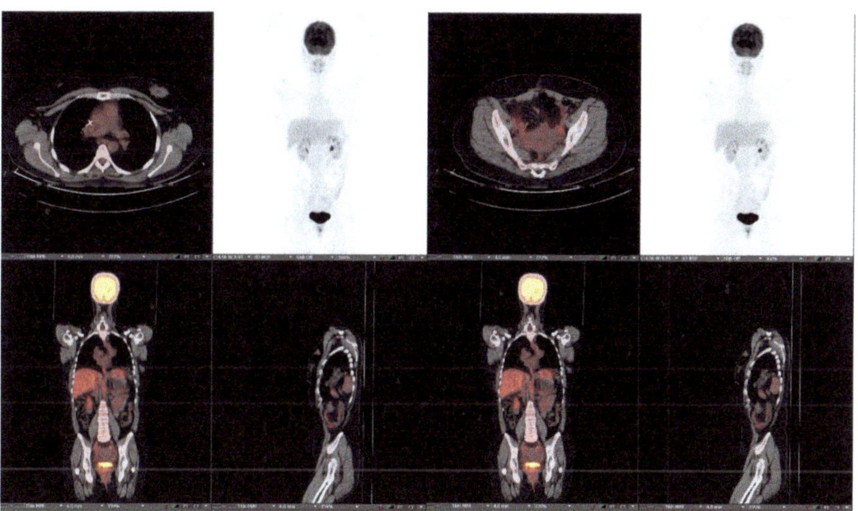

References

Jung Y, Tae KTH, Kim JY, et al. The effect of sex hormones on normal breast tissue metabolism. Evaluation by FDG PET/CT. Medicine. 2019;98:27.

Kim TH, Kim MR, Jung Y, et al. Relationship between sex hormones levels and F-18 FDG uptake by the ovaries in premenopausal woman. Radiol Oncol. 2019;53(3):293–9.

Chapter 17
Case 17: Rising PSA in Radical Prostatectomy for Prostate Cancer

A: PET and bone scans in an 82-year-old man post radical prostatectomy 23 years ago with rising PSA 4.72 (2 months ago) from 2.14 (4 months ago) while on androgen deprivation therapy. (1) What are the tracers? (2) Is there any evidence of bone metastasis? (3) How is PET scanning done? (4) Where is the most intense activity in the normal bio-distribution of this PET tracer? (5) What is the reference SUV in the PET?

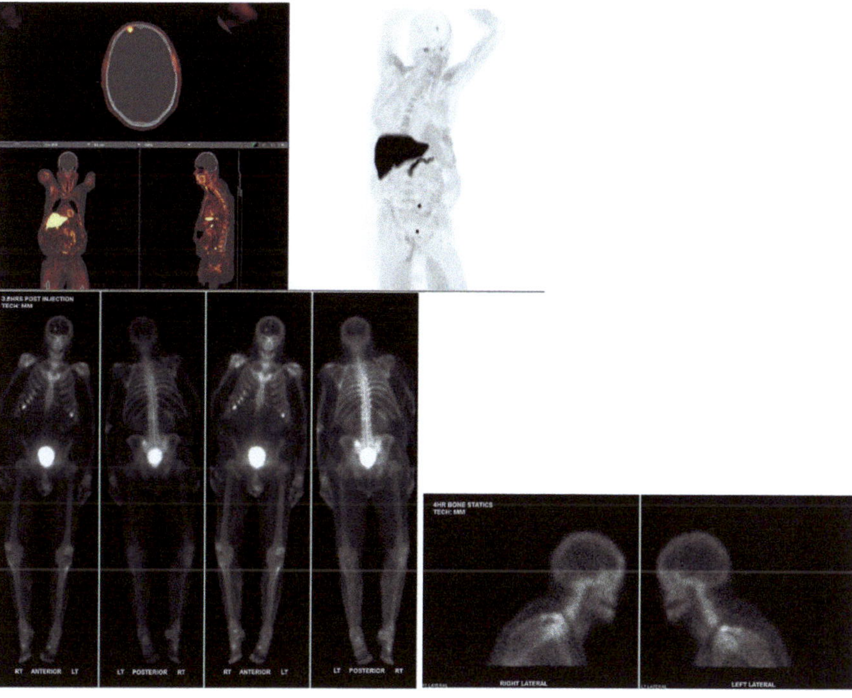

C. Y. O. Wong, D. Wu, *Phenotypic Oncology PET*,
https://doi.org/10.1007/978-3-031-09737-9_17

B: Transverse slices of PET in the abdomen and pelvis. (1) What is (are) the additional finding(s)? (2) What's the appropriate recommendation on scanning and regional normalization?

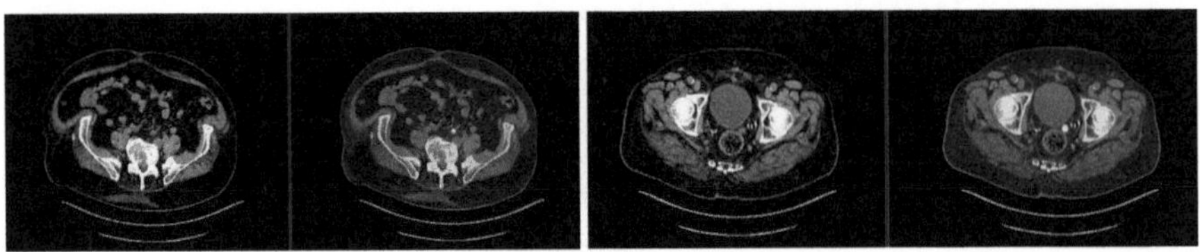

17.1 Case 17: Interpretation and Teaching

A1: F-18 fluciclovine and Tc-99 MDP.

A2: A small 2–3 mm lytic lesion in the right side of the skull is avid SUV 5.08 where it appears to have an asymmetric uptake by the recent bone scan, indicating bone metastatic disease.

Teaching Point 1 Although the lesion is positive in both PET and bone scan in the right frontal skull, the former is more sensitive than the latter. Fluciclovine PET can also evaluate the soft tissue metastasis, being more sensitive than FDG PET where tumor may be of low metabolic phenotype.

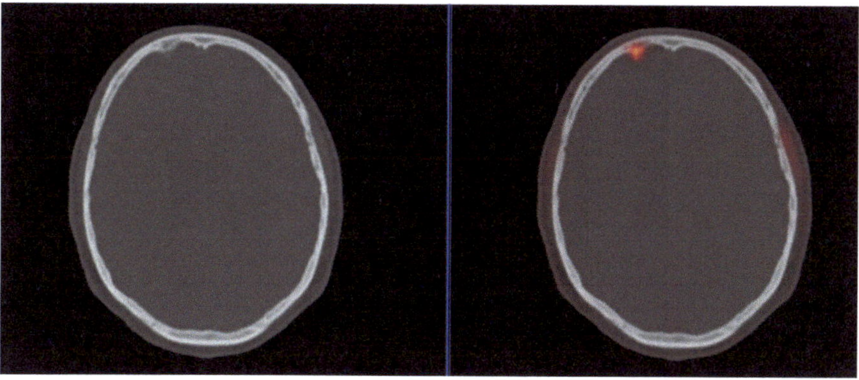

A3: Approximately 2.5 min after the intravenous administration of 10.4 mCi of Axumin (18F-fluciclovine), PET emission images and CT transmission images were acquired from the proximal thighs to the top of the head, in the reverse direction of FDG PET to bypass the urine collection in the GU system.

A4: Physiologic uptake is most intense in the liver and pancreas. Physiologic uptake in the marrow is mild.

A5: Reference: 1.0 cm blood pool mean SUV is 1.17 and 1.5 cm L3 marrow mean SUV is 2.34.

B1: Prior radical prostatectomy bed showed no evidence of avid recurrent or residual mass. However posterior to the bladder on the left is avid (SUV 16.22) small nodule measuring 1.4 cm that is suggestive of metastatic disease. Another avid (SUV 16.72) metastatic lymph node is seen at left common iliac region measuring 1.4 × 1.1 cm.

B2: Thus, due to high liver uptake, assessment of abdominal and pelvic areas may need some regional normalization.

Teaching Point 2 If a focal avid lesion or homogenous diffuse uptake has SUV greater than marrow, it is positive. If a focal avid lesion smaller than 1 cm or has heterogeneous diffuse uptake greater than blood pool, it is positive.

Reference

Chen B, Wei P, Macapinlac HA, et al. Comparison of 18F-Fluciclovine PET/CT and 99mTc-MDP bone scan in detection of bone metastasis in prostate cancer. Nucl Med Commun. 2019;40(9):940–6.

Chapter 18
Case 18: Concurrent Lung and Brain Metastatic Cancer

A: Restaging PET (left panel) for a 78-year-old with history of stage IIIB distal esophageal invasive moderately differentiated adenocarcinoma (right panel baseline PET 4 months ago) status post-chemoradiation, esophagectomy, partial gastrectomy, gastric pull-through, adjuvant chemotherapy, and prior heavy smoking having slightly growing bilateral lung nodules by CT further diagnosis. (1) What is the tracer? (2) Is the uptake on the nodule in the right middle lobe (RML) significant for new second primary cancer or metastasis?

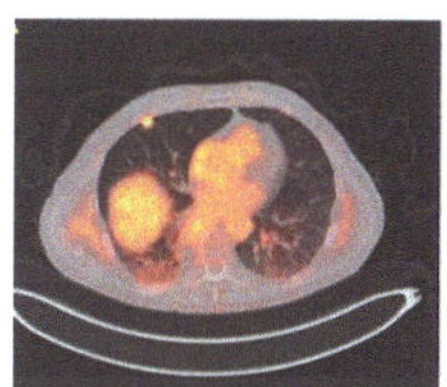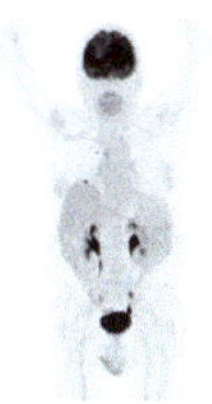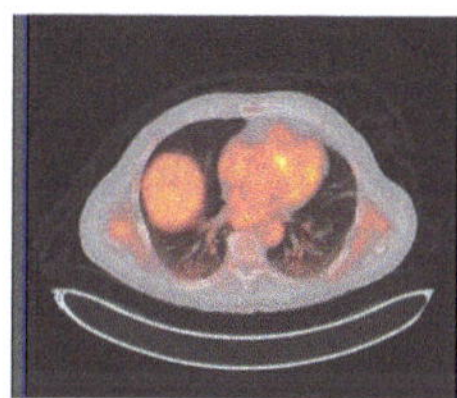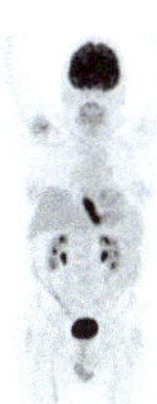

B: Current brain image (left) with subsequent MRI (middle) and prior brain PET (right). (1) What is the likely etiology of the "apparently non-avid" focus relative to the rest of brain metabolism in the parietal lobe? (2) Is the avid RML lung nodule related to this diagnosis?

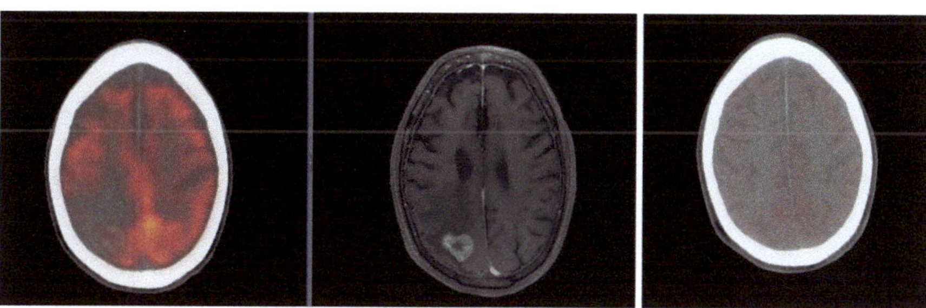

18.1   Case 18: Interpretation and Teaching

A1:   F-18 FDG.

A2:   Although the most avid one in the right middle lobe measuring 12 mm has SUV 10.11, there are many new scattered small bilateral pleural- and parenchymal-based nodules that are noted with avidity in varying degrees, for instance, in the right upper lobe (left panel compared to baseline PET on right panel) compatible with metastatic disease rather than second primary tumor.

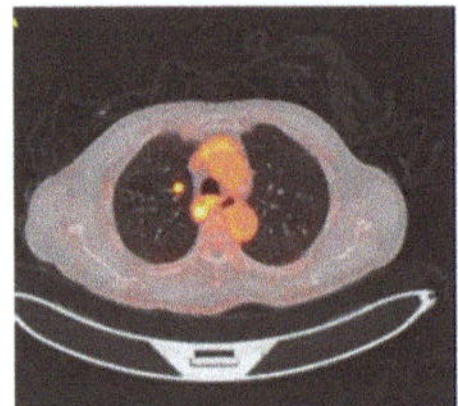 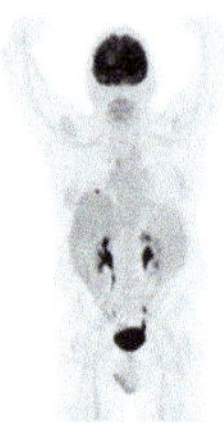 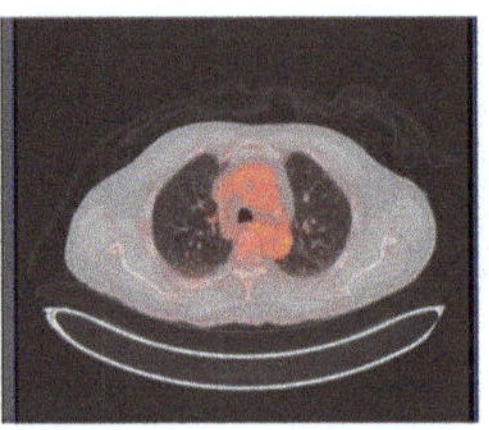 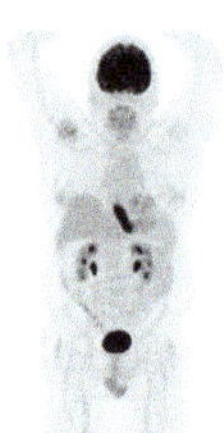

B1:   A 1.5 cm roundish lesion is seen on CT with hyperdense rim which is new from old PET-CT associated with adjacent hypometabolism (SUV 6.9 compared to the contralateral SUV 9.54; right cerebellar SUV 9.58) in the right parietal region suspicious of metastasis with edema or mass effects. There is no abnormal uptake in the rest of the head and neck, including the larynx and thyroid gland. Subsequent brain MRI confirmed single metastasis and craniotomy showed metastatic adenocarcinoma.

B2:   The initial avid thickening of distal esophagus extending into the fundus from original primary malignancy (SUV 19.07) has been treated and resected. Since there is evidence of lung metastasis as exemplified by the avid RML nodule, the brain diagnosis is related to the same neoplastic process.

Teaching Point   Only about 70% of brain metastases appear to be avid relatively to the adjacent neuronal activity. Thus, the evaluation of brain metastasis by FDG PET is very limited. Inclusion of the brain routinely in whole-body F-FDG PET-CT studies detected previously unknown metastases in less than 1%, impacting insignificantly the PET staging. MRI shall be recommended if there is any clinical suspicion for complete staging.

Reference

Manohar K, Bhattacharya A, Mittal BR. Low positive yield from routine inclusion of the brain in whole-body 18F-FDG PET/CT imaging for noncerebral malignancies: results from a large population study. Nucl Med Commun. 2013;34(6):540–3.

Chapter 19
Case 19: Tumor Phenotypes in Metastatic Prostate Cancer

A: Restaging PET in a 68-year-old with prostate cancer status post-robotic-assisted radical prostatectomy and lymph node sampling to be pathologically T3bN0 and local radiation 6 years ago and Lupron injection. Another PET 11 months ago showed bone metastasis and obstructive right hydronephrosis status post-nephrostomy tube on Xtandi with PSA persistently rising up switching to Zytiga/prednisone for current treatment. (1) What are the tracers? (2) What are the PET findings on the bony structures? (3) Is the tumor load on bone congruent in both PET scans?

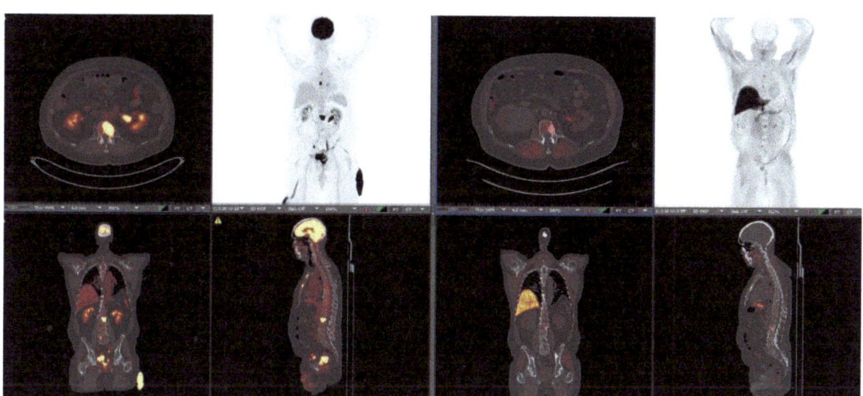

C. Y. O. Wong, D. Wu, *Phenotypic Oncology PET*,
https://doi.org/10.1007/978-3-031-09737-9_19

B: Soft tissue window PET images. (1) What is the likely etiology of the avid focus in the pelvis? (2) Is the avid lesion related to urinary obstruction?

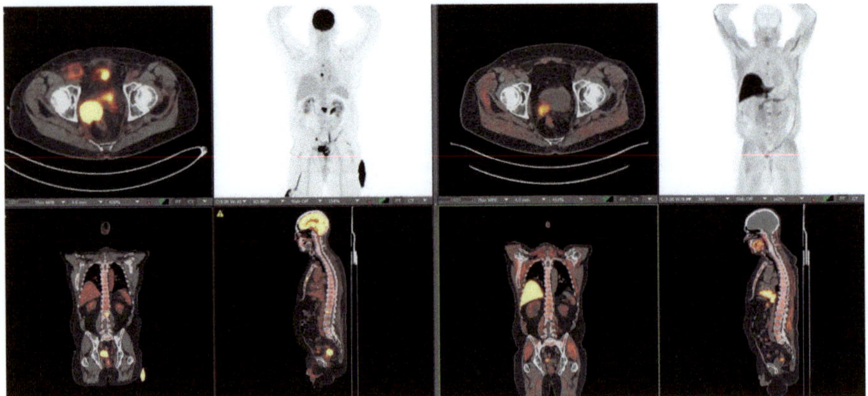

19.1 Case 19: Interpretation and Teaching

A1: F-18 FDG and F-18 fluciclovine for left and right panels of PET images.

A2 and A3: Multiple avid mixed lytic and sclerotic lesions are seen in the skeleton consistent with metastatic disease, and many of these demonstrate congruent avid activity as in the following table and graph (PSA in ng/ml):

Lesion #	Tracer	FDG	Fluciclovine	
	PSA	2.94	0.84	
	TX	ZYTIGA	XTANDI	In (FDG SUV)
1	Manubrium	3.8	3.6	1.333
2	Sternum	20.7	5.8	3.030
3	L2	26.9	6.4	3.292
4	L5	3.6	4.3	1.267
5	Right ilium	2.9	3.1	1.068

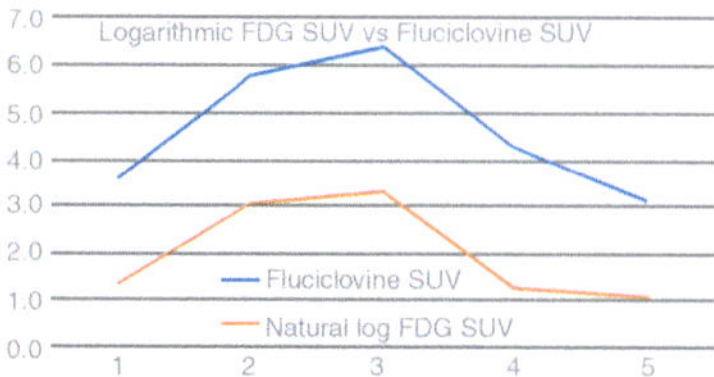

B1 and B2: There is 36 × 45 mm avid soft tissue density in region of distal right ureter/UVJ with FDG SUV 29.81 compared to radioactive urine in bladder SUV 13.55 with Foley catheter in place. The prior moderate to marked hydronephrosis and hydroureter on the right were relieved by percutaneous nephrostomy tube, and the fluciclovine SUV of the same lesion was 5.69 with urine SUV 0.76.

Reference SUV in mediastinal blood pool and normal L3 marrow for FDG versus fluciclovine were 2.14 and 2.43 versus 1.14 and 3.4, respectively.

C: Bone window PET-CT showed sclerotic lesion still having avid uptake in both tracers.

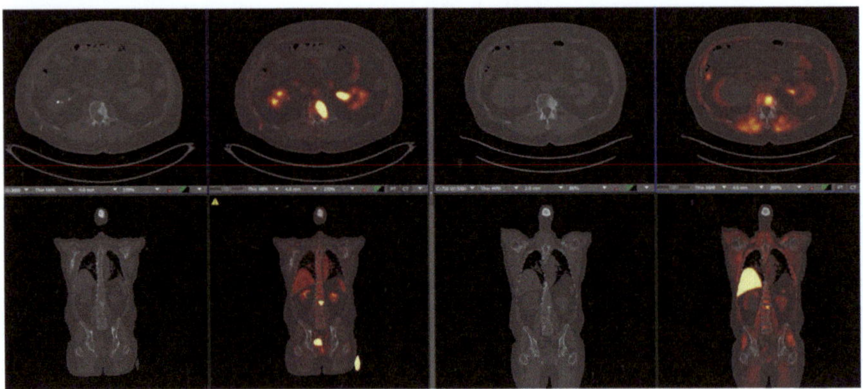

Teaching Point The sclerotic lesions in metastatic lesions from prostate cancer may be still active, unlike those in other cancers which usually represent healing after treatment. The ultimate healing requires negative results on bone scan (F-18 NaF or Tc-99m MDP).

Reference

O'Sullivan GJ, Carty FL, Cronin CG. Imaging of bone metastasis: an update. World J Radiol. 2015;7(8):202–11.

Chapter 20
Case 20: Metastatic Recurrent Melanoma

A: Restaging PET-CT (left panel) was performed on this 49-year-old female with history of malignant melanoma right third toe (stage IIIA) with right inguinal/femoral nodal metastases status post-wide local excision lymph node dissection (3 years ago) and adjuvant immunotherapy (Opdivo). Right medial thigh melanoma received wide local excision without residual disease 15 months ago. Last PET (right panel) 6 months ago was negative with immunotherapy completed 15 months before the PET. (1) What is the tracer? (2) What's the PET diagnosis? (3) What is the next step of management?

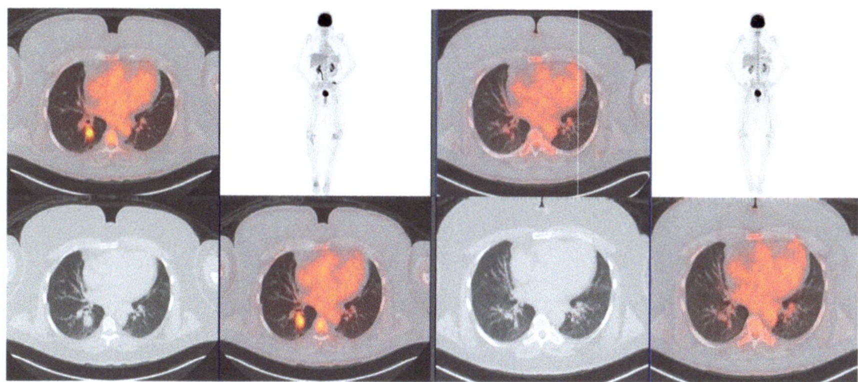

© The Author(s), under exclusive license to Springer Nature
Switzerland AG 2022
C. Y. O. Wong, D. Wu, *Phenotypic Oncology PET*,
https://doi.org/10.1007/978-3-031-09737-9_20

20.1   Case 20: Interpretation and Teaching

A1:   F-18 FDG.

A2:   A new right lower lung avid mass is noted with SUV 4.12 at 28 × 20 mm by CT which is suspicious of metastatic malignancy, focal pneumonia, or rapidly growing primary lung cancer.

A3:   Further evaluation by short-term dedicated contrast CT chest or tissue correlation is suggested.

B: CT-guided biopsy (left image) showed poorly differentiated spindle and epithelioid neoplasm, not excluding metastatic melanoma. As BRAF V600E was weak positive, therapy begun with dabrafenib and trametinib. There was interval decrease in size of right lower lobe metastatic melanoma by CT 2 months apart. The CT images of pretherapy (right most) and 1 month after therapy (middle posttherapy) are shown.

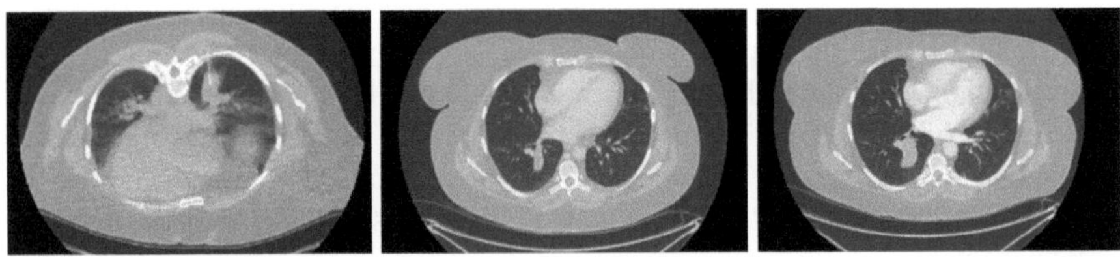

Teaching Point Melanoma workup needs whole-body PET-CT, and recurrent or metastatic melanoma is usually FDG avid, and negative PET has high predictive value of being in remission.

Reference

Vensby PH, Schmidt G, Kjær A, et al. The value of FDG PET/CT for follow-up of patients with melanoma: a retrospective analysis. Am J Nucl Med Mol Imaging. 2017;7(6):255–62.

Chapter 21
Case 21: Post-prostatectomy for Prostate Cancer with Rising PSA

A: PET imaging for Gleason 10 prostate carcinoma with bone, lymph node, and brain metastases on olaparib 300 mg bid po with Lupron-Xgeva injections at 3 month intervals. Biopsy-proven brain metastases were treated by gamma knife stereotactic radiosurgery on dexamethasone. Restaging with rising PSA (9.34 ng/ml 1 month ago and 1.67 ng/ml 5 months ago). Left panel is current PET; right panel is prior PET. (1) What is the tracer? (2) What do you see in the prostate region? (3) What are the interval references?

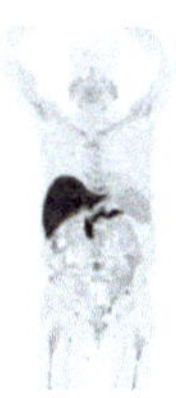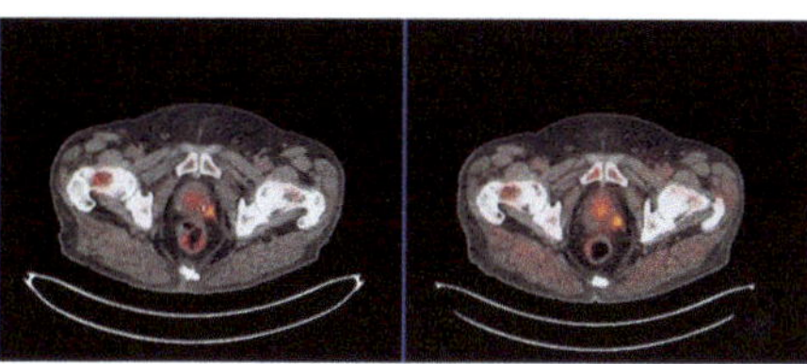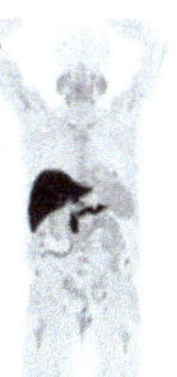

B: PET images of the brain after (left) and before (right) gamma knife therapy. (1) Is there a response or recurrence? (2) What is the tracer to differentiate radionecrosis or recurrence?

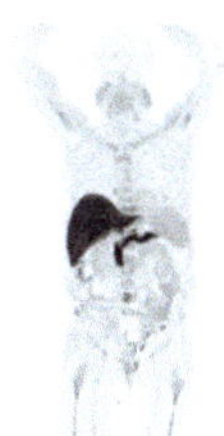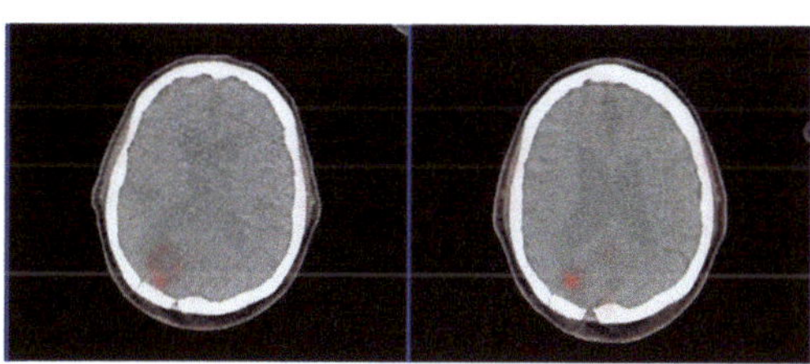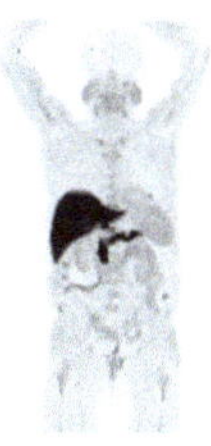

C. Y. O. Wong, D. Wu, *Phenotypic Oncology PET*,
https://doi.org/10.1007/978-3-031-09737-9_21

C: PET images of the chest after (top left first and third) and before (top left second and fourth images) treatment together with bones after (bottom left two images) and before (bottom right two images) therapy. (1) Is there a progression? (2) What are other imaging modalities needed?

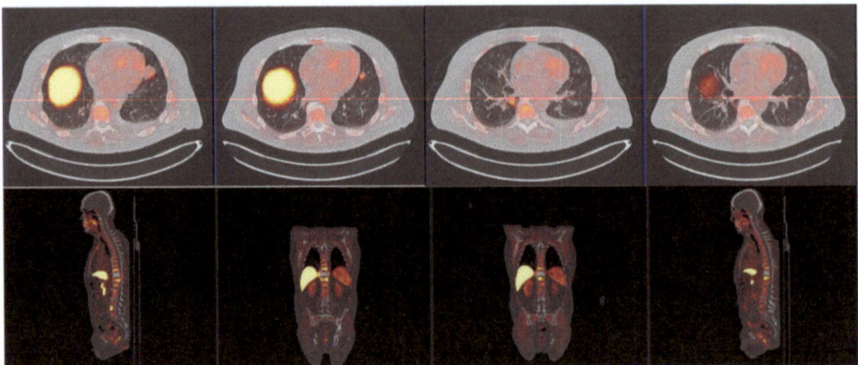

21.1   Case 21: Interpretation and Teaching

A1:   F-18 fluciclovine.

A2:   There is stable neoplastic process in the prostate region by fluciclovine; SUV maximum at the periphery of the prostate fossa left of midline is 5.26 compared to (cf) 4.73 and in the central prostate fossa is 3.81 cf 3.88.

A3:   The internal references (cf=compared to prior PET) are 1.0 cm blood pool mean SUV 1.50 cf 1.54 and 1.5 cm L3 marrow mean SUV 2.75 cf 2.67.

B1:   The previously reported 9 × 4 mm lesion in the right occipital white matter (by MRI) has been treated with peripheral rim of active SUV 2.55 and centrally necrotic SUV 1.05 cf prior solid mass 2.95. There is adjacent 13 × 5 mm dural-based right parietal-temporal mass which has SUV 2.90 cf 4.59. Treated brain metastasis shows central necrosis but there is peripheral avidity. The adjacent dural-based right parietal-temporal seeding has also decreased uptake (left cf right PET-CT). Some response is likely.

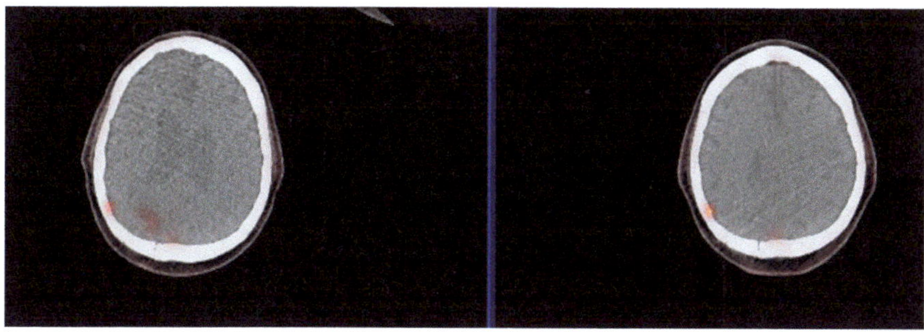

B2:   It may be evaluated by FDG PET for radionecrosis versus residual tumor. Correlation with gamma knife RTP map and further evaluation by brain MRI for other potential brain metastasis are recommended.

Teaching Point Using a SUV_{max} threshold of ≥ 1.3, Fluciclovine PET demonstrated a 100% accuracy in distinguishing recurrent disease from radiation necrosis up to 30 min after injection. However, tumor-to-background ratios (TBR_{max}) were not significantly different between recurrent disease and radiation necrosis at any time point due to variable levels of fluciclovine uptake in the background brain parenchyma.

C1:   There is progression of metastasis in lungs and bones, and PSA has increased from date of prior PET to current PET at a level of 4.53 ng/ml.

C2:   As there are sclerosis without avid uptake, bone scan may be helpful to document healing or eroding.

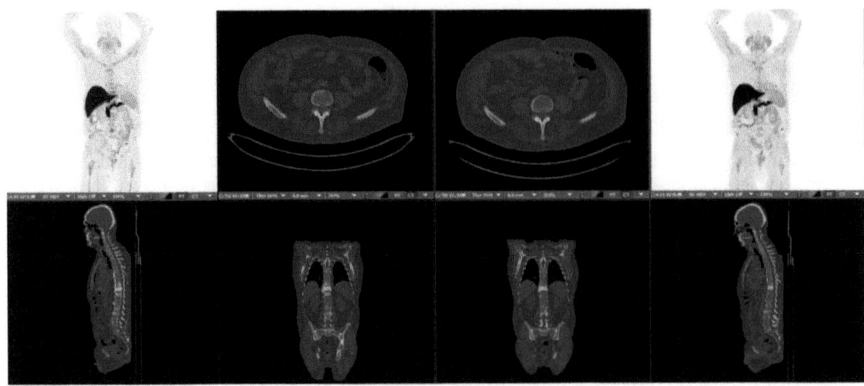

Reference

Parent EE, Patel D, Nye JA, et al. [18F]-Fluciclovine PET discrimination of recurrent intracranial metastatic disease from radiation necrosis. EJNMMI Res. 2020;10, Article number: 148

Chapter 22
Case 22: Left Adrenal Mass

A: PET imaging for left adrenal mass for diagnosis and/or staging. (1) What is the tracer? (2) What is normal distribution? (3) What do you see in the adrenal regions? (4) What is the diagnosis?

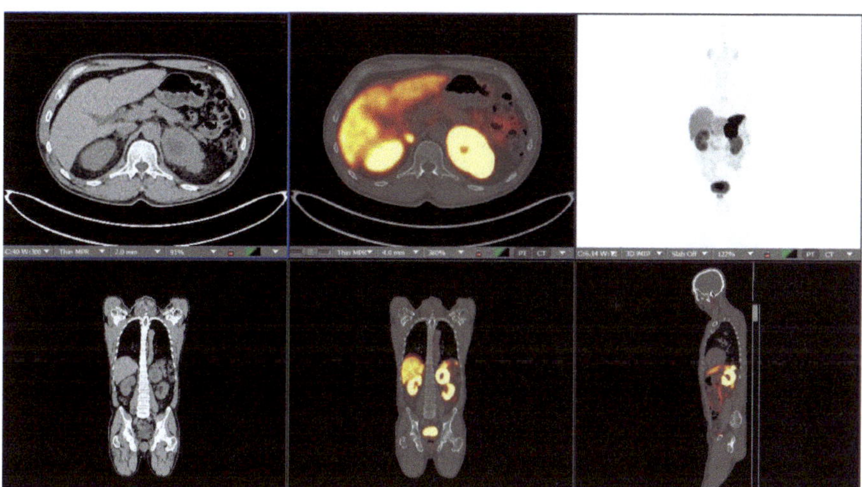

© The Author(s), under exclusive license to Springer Nature
Switzerland AG 2022

C. Y. O. Wong, D. Wu, *Phenotypic Oncology PET*,
https://doi.org/10.1007/978-3-031-09737-9_22

B: PET images of the sternum. (1) Is there a metastasis or other diagnosis? (2) What is uptake at the sternoclavicular junction?

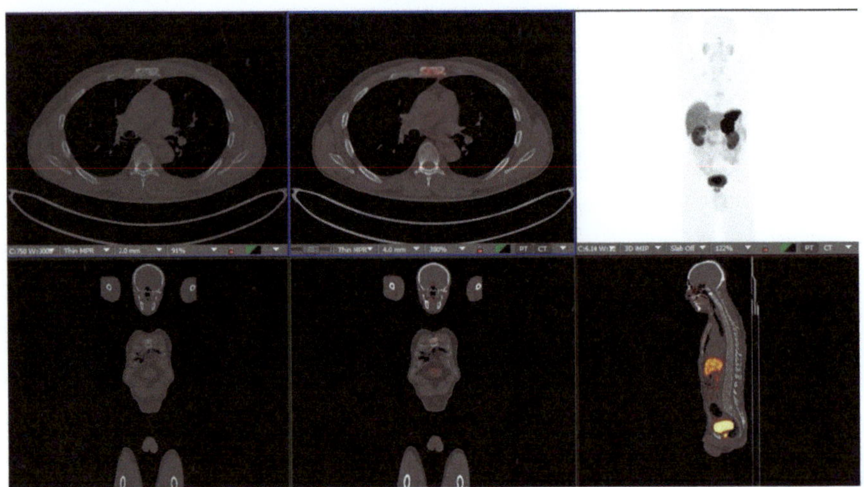

22.1 Case 22: Interpretation and Teaching

A1:   Cu-64 DOTATATE (3.6 mCi administered intravenously with 64 min uptake).

A2:   There is normal uptake in the spleen, liver, and endocrine glands.

A3:   There is normal physiologic uptake at right adrenal gland (SUV 8.86), but there is large centrally necrotic/cavitary left adrenal mass measuring 70×53 mm in the axial plane with SUV 49.4.

A4:   Left adrenal pheochromocytoma.

B1:   Mild activity fusing to the sternum has SUV 2.9 compatible with healing fracture as there is similar uptake in the rib fractures such as the right first rib (SUV 2.09).

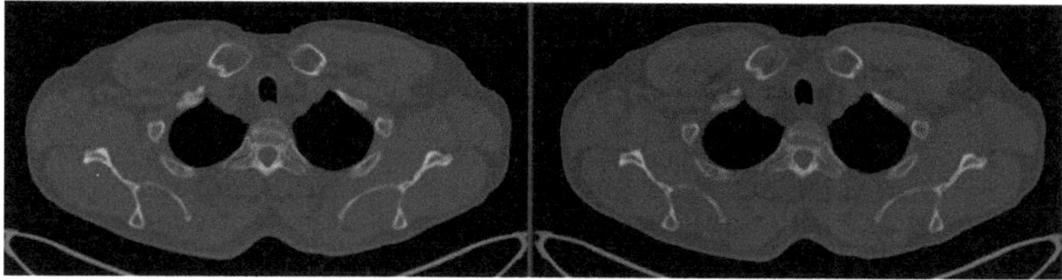

B2:   It is from osteoarthritic changes (SUV at left side 2.31).

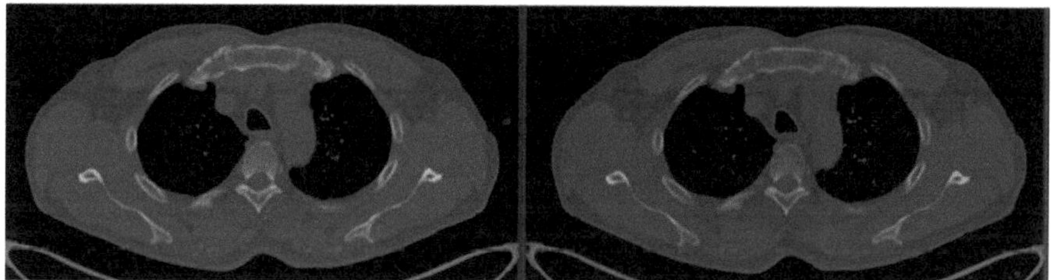

Teaching Point ^{64}Cu-DOTATATE PET-CT imaging 1–3 h after injection is excellent for lesion detection in patients with neuroendocrine neoplasms (NENs) due to longer half-life at 12.7 h than that of ^{68}Ga-DOTATATE at 68 min. Both tracers have avid uptake in the pheochromocytoma. The uptake in the bones is too low to be metastasis and it is from inflammation.

Reference

Loft M, Carlsen EA, Johnbeck CB, et al. ^{64}Cu-DOTATATE PET in patients with neuroendocrine neoplasms: prospective, head-to-head comparison of imaging at 1 hour and 3 hours after injection. J Nucl Med 2021, 62 (1): 73-80.

Chapter 23
Case 23: Cutaneous T-Cell Lymphoma

A: PET imaging for skin lesion at left back for diagnosis and/or staging. (1) What is the tracer? (2) Is uptake typical for cutaneous lymphoma?

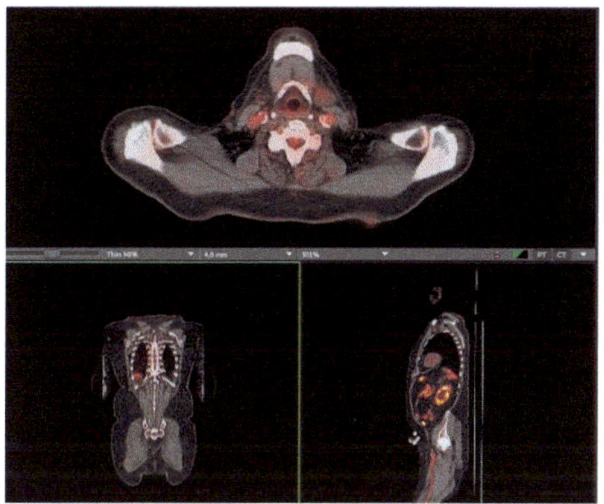 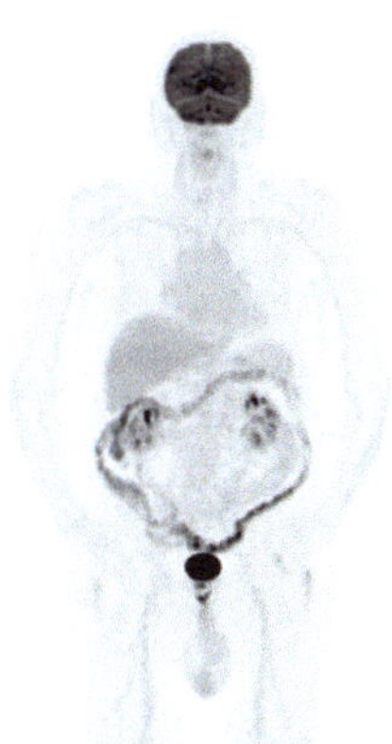

C. Y. O. Wong, D. Wu, *Phenotypic Oncology PET*,
https://doi.org/10.1007/978-3-031-09737-9_23

23.1   Case 23: Interpretation and Teaching

A1:   F-18 FDG.
A2:   There is usually low uptake in cutaneous lymphoma. This is from an 81-year-old man with T-cell CD4-positive cutaneous lymphoma favoring mycosis fungoides on biopsy.

Teaching Point   Primary cutaneous lymphoma (PCL) is the second most common type of extranodal non-Hodgkin's lymphoma, including both cutaneous T-cell and B-cell lymphomas. Although F-FDG PET and PET-CT have relatively low uptake and do not seem to adequately distinguish the plaque, patch, or erythroderma cutaneous lesions of PCL, the imaging modalities are superior to CT, MRI, and other nuclear medicine methods in detecting both the cutaneous and the extracutaneous lesions of PCL. Clinically it is promising in staging, tumor biological evaluation, biopsy guidance, early treatment response assessment, and recurrence surveillance.

Reference

Qiu L, Tu G, Li J, et al. The role of 18F-FDG PET and PET/CT in the evaluation of primary cutaneous lymphoma. Nucl Med Commun. 2017;38(2):106–16.

Chapter 24
Case 24: Active Myeloma Versus Schmorl's Node

A: This is a 39-years-old female with monoclonal paraproteinemia (smoldering myeloma from recent bone marrow diagnosis, MGUS) for restaging. (1) What is tracer? (2) Is uptake at active myeloma or Schmorl's node at L2? (3) Is there any abnormal uptake at bones? (4) What other imaging is suggested for differentiation?

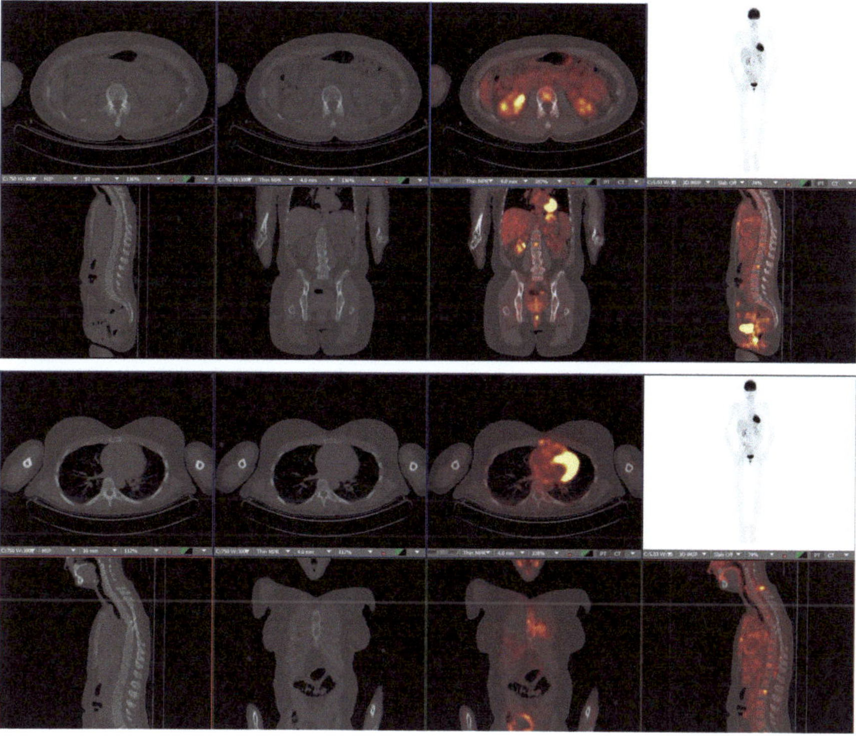

C. Y. O. Wong, D. Wu, *Phenotypic Oncology PET*,
https://doi.org/10.1007/978-3-031-09737-9_24

24.1   Case 24: Interpretation and Teaching

A1:   F-18 FDG

A2 and A3:   Focal uptake is noted at a lucent area of L2 posterior vertebral body with SUV 4.66. Focal uptake is also noted at the mid sternum with SUV 3.67 without detectable bone lesion. The reference mediastinal blood pool SUV is 1.53 and marrow SUV at L3 is 2.15. There is inflammatory uptake in the spinous process of C6 (SUV 5.03). Focal uptake at lucent area of L2 may be Schmorl's node or myeloma. But there is a sternal uptake favoring active myeloma.

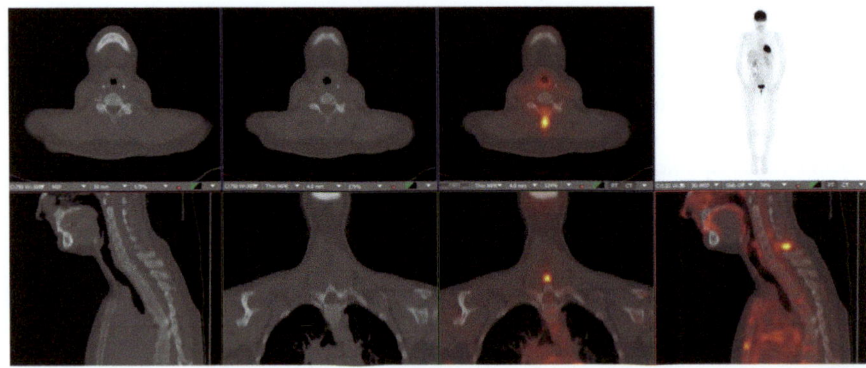

A4:   Further evaluation by MRI is helpful. Since the prior MRI of the lumbar spine about two and half years ago, there has been development of an approximately 12 × 11 mm T1 hypointense (left image), STIR hyperintense (right image) and mildly enhancing lesion (middle image) within the posterior aspect of the L2 vertebral body, and thus the lesion is suspicious for myelomatous lesion given the history and the interval development of the lesion.

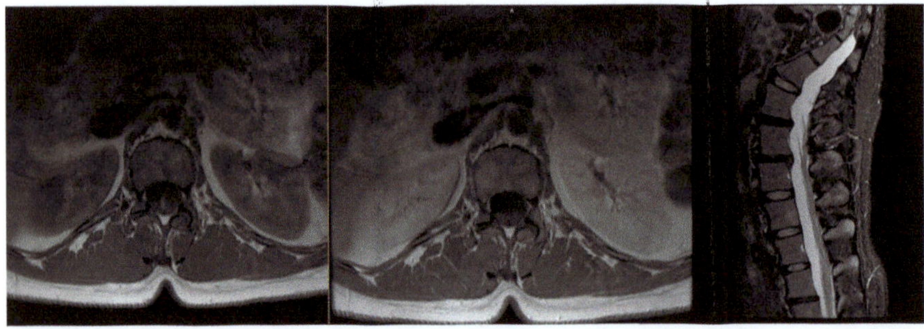

Teaching Point There has been remarkable progress made in the diagnosis and treatment of multiple myeloma (MM). PET-CT is used to diagnose MM bone disease and allow the initiation of effective therapy to prevent the development of end-organ damage for patients who are at the highest risk.

Reference

Rajkumar SV. Updated diagnostic criteria and staging system for multiple myeloma. Am Soc Clin Oncol Educ Book. 2016;35:e418–23.

Chapter 25
Case 25: Small-Cell Lung Cancer

A: This is a 68-year-old female with history of bilateral breast malignancies and right primary pulmonary neuroendocrine tumor (rightmost panel) with ischial-anal metastasis post-chemoradiation 5 months ago for restaging (left two panels for subsequent follow-up). (1) What are the tracers? (2) Is uptake at right apex from active residual tumor or postradiation changes? (3) Is there any abnormal uptake at mediastinal node? (4) What other PET imaging is suggested for differentiation?

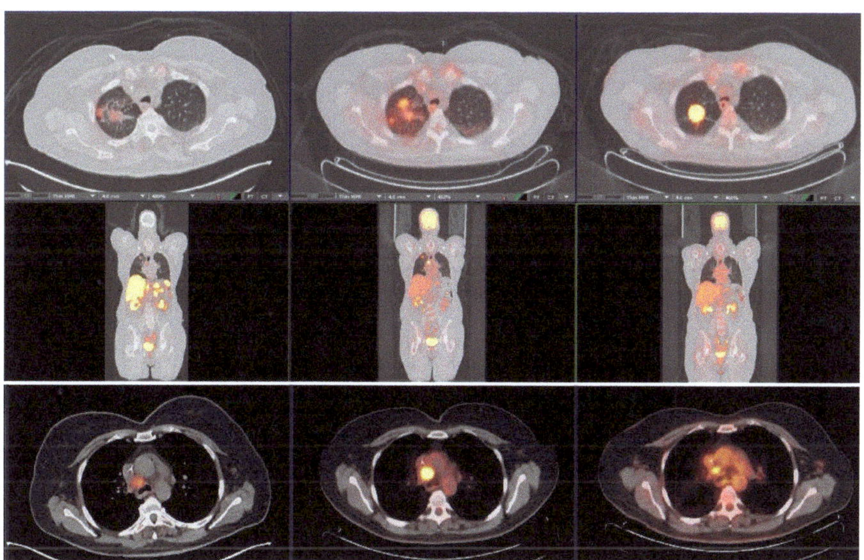

© The Author(s), under exclusive license to Springer Nature
Switzerland AG 2022
C. Y. O. Wong, D. Wu, *Phenotypic Oncology PET*,
https://doi.org/10.1007/978-3-031-09737-9_25

B: Subsequent two additional PET imaging were done 7.5 (leftmost), 6.5 (middle), and 5 (rightmost) months after chemoradiation. (1) What are the tracers? (2) Is breast uptake from recurrence breast cancer or metastasis? (3) What is etiology of avid uptake in mediastinal node? (4) What is etiology of avid uptake in right apex? (5) What is overall response to chemotherapy?

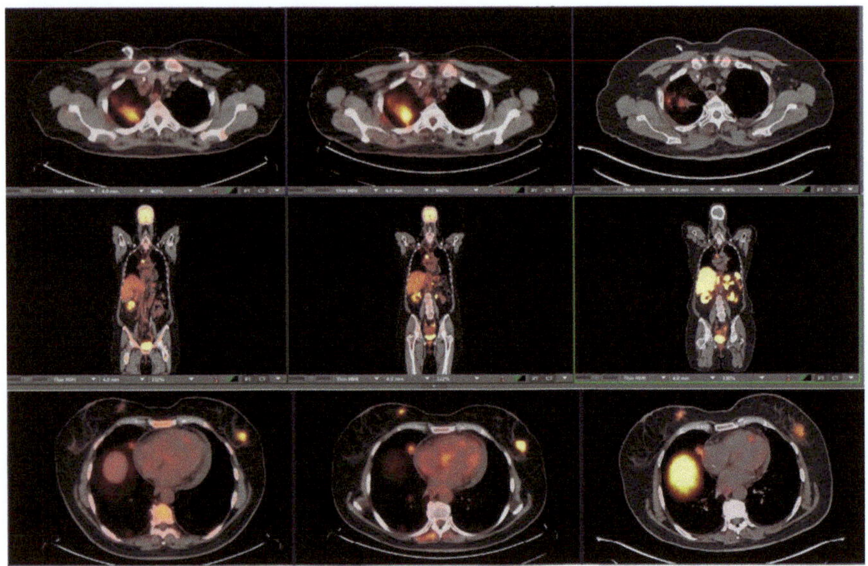

25.1   Case 25: Interpretation and Teaching

A1:   F-18 FDG, F-18 FDG and Ga-68 DOTA-Tyr-octreotate (DOTATATE) from right to left panels.

A2:   Right upper lobe cancer was estimated at 2.3 × 2.5 mm with SUV 12.87 after chemotherapy compared to prior 2.9 × 2.5 cm with SUV maximum 12.35. After radiation, the FDG SUV was 3.2 with diffuse pneumonitis with DOTA SUV 3.03.

A3 and A4:   There is right lower paratracheal node increased FDG uptake SUV 10.34 (3.86, previously before radiation) with DOTA SUV 3.86, suggesting inflammation.

Teaching Point   There has been discrepancy between FDG and DOTA uptake in nodal area suggesting likely inflammation as the primary cancer has concordant uptake after radiation.

B1:   F-18 FDG, F-18 FDG and Ga-68 DOTA-Tyr-octreotate (DOTATATE) from right to left panels.

B2:   There are again multiple hypermetabolic nodular densities within the breast tissues bilaterally. The 2.2 × 1.5 cm density within the right inferior breast has SUV 6.32 (8.6 previously; DOTA SUV 3.89). On the left side, the 2.4 × 2.0 cm nodular density laterally has SUV 5.27 (7.0 previously; DOTA SUV 3.58) which was likely metastatic lung neuroendocrine tumor.

B3:   There is a persistent enlarged, markedly hypermetabolic right precarinal lymph node, which measures approximately 1.7 × 1.6 cm with SUV 7.78 (2.0 × 1.7 cm with SUV 10.1 previously; DOTA SUV 3.86), consistent with inflammation though a residual mediastinal nodal metastasis cannot be excluded.

B4:   The right apical opacity 3.2 × 1.7 cm has SUV 4.16 (4.8 × 3.4 cm with SUV 5.8 previously; DOTA SUV 3.03), likely radiation pneumonitis.

B5:   The patient has other metastasis besides in the liver, omentum, abdominal nodes, and bones. Thus, there is extrapulmonary progression since DOTA scan where the intensity in the liver has been adjusted down.

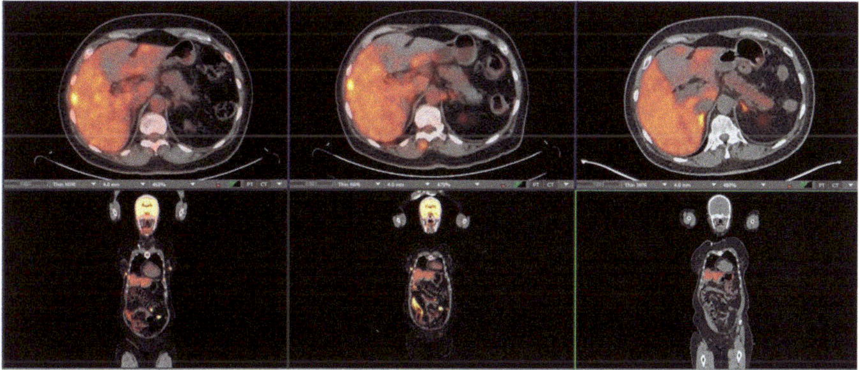

Teaching Point Low-grade neuroendocrine tumors showed significantly higher uptake of DOTATATE and significantly less uptake of FDG than did tumors of higher grade. There was no instance of false-positive uptake of DOTATATE secondary to inflammation. Inflammatory uptake is invariably low grade in postradiation therapy change.

Reference

Kayani I, Conry BG, Groves AM, et al. A comparison of 68Ga-DOTATATE and 18F-FDG PET/CT in pulmonary neuroendocrine tumors. J Nucl Med. 2009;50(12):1927–32.

Chapter 26
Case 26: Synchronous PEComa and Lung Adenocarcinoma

A: This is an 85-year-old female with left breast cancer post-lumpectomy and radiation 34 years ago for restaging. SBRT (stereotactic body radiation therapy) for right upper lung adenocarcinoma (adenoCA) completed 4 months ago for restaging. In the left two-column panels are post-SBRT images. In the right two-column panels are baseline PET images. (1) What are the tracers? (2) Is uptake at the upper abdomen a metastasis or synchronous second tumor? (3) What is the response in the lung cancer? (4) What is malignant potential of the upper abdomen?

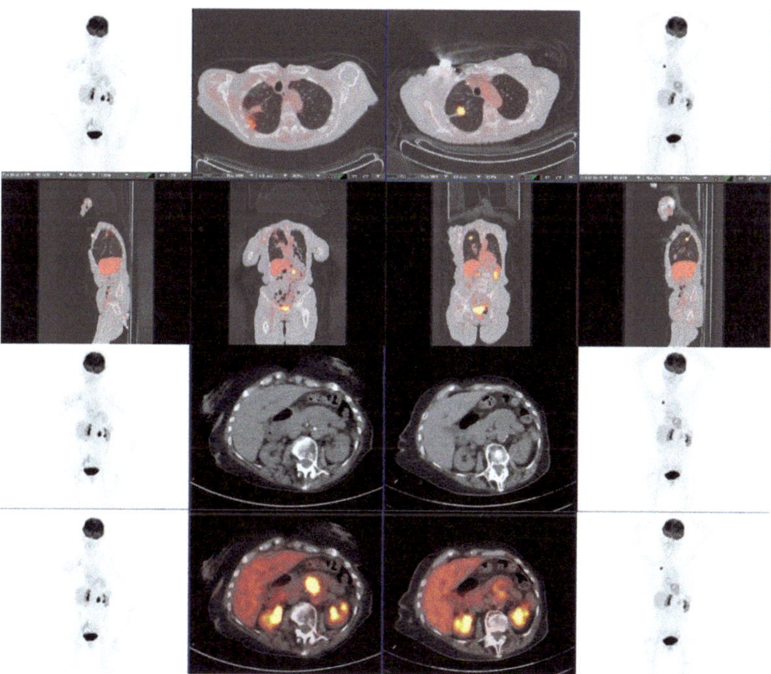

C. Y. O. Wong, D. Wu, *Phenotypic Oncology PET*,
https://doi.org/10.1007/978-3-031-09737-9_26

26.1   Case 26: Interpretation and Teaching

A1:   Both are F-18 FDG.

A2:   The 31 × 30 mm necrotic mass found to be the perivascular epithelioid cell tumor (PEComa) just posterior to pancreas and anterior to the aorta with associated peripheral avid activity and maximum SUV 4.0 becomes more solid and avid on medial aspect with SUV 16.58, but it is stable in size at 31 × 20 mm.

A3:   Prior FDG-avid 29 × 18 mm right upper lobe adenocarcinoma with SUV 11.4, abutting major fissure, has been irradiated with SUV 2.10 at 14 × 11 mm density with postradiation pneumonitis, suggesting good response.

A4:   Prior FDG-avid necrotic PEComa anterior to the aorta has been markedly increasing avidity for which malignant potential is suspected. The CT portion usually shows a necrotic lesion to enhance in the delayed phase (sequence of images: pre-contrast, arterial, and venous phase).

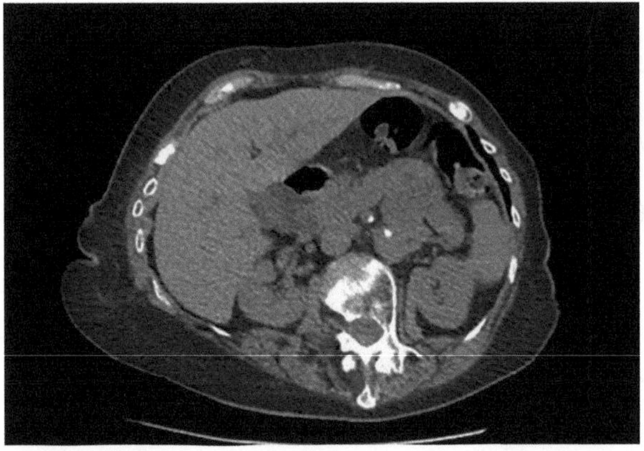

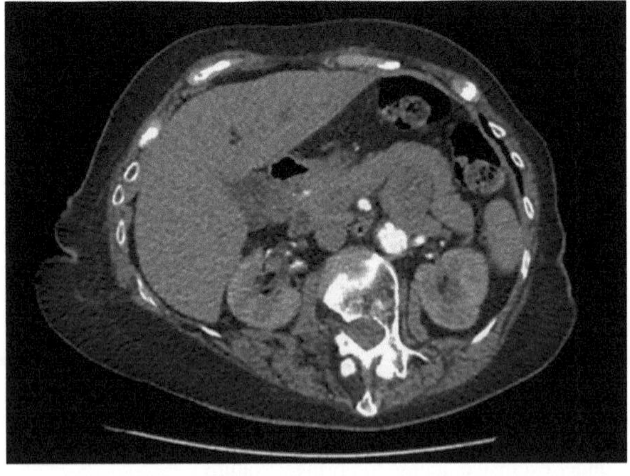

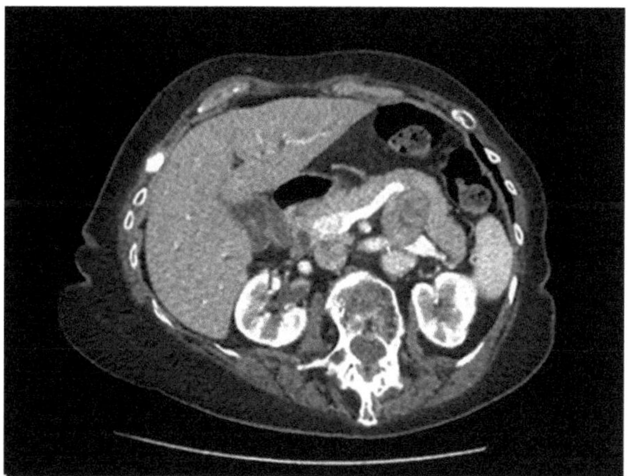

Teaching Point
1. Prior FDG-avid right upper lobe nodule adenoCA has been treated by SBRT with large reduction of metabolism great than 60% indicating good response. The postradiation pneumonitis may be peaking around 8 months later.
2. PEComa is a rare tumor with varying malignant potential. PEComas have a wide variety of presentations and behavior. Reports have suggested that criteria for malignancy include tumor greater than 5 cm, mitotic rate of more than 1 per 50 high-power field, and necrosis, but this has not been universally adopted. The change to higher metabolism raises concern of malignant potential.

Chapter 27
Case 27: Breast Cancer After Immunochemotherapy

A: The patient is 66-years-old with metastatic right breast cancer to axillary lymph nodes status post-excision, radiation therapy, and systemic treatment (Carbo/Gemzar/Keytruda, cycle 2) for restaging. Left panel (two left columns of images in two chest sections) shows post-immunochemotherapy and right panel (two right columns) shows the baseline images. (1) What is the tracer? (2) Is the new uptake at mediastinum progression of metastasis? (3) What is the response of the breast cancer metastasis?

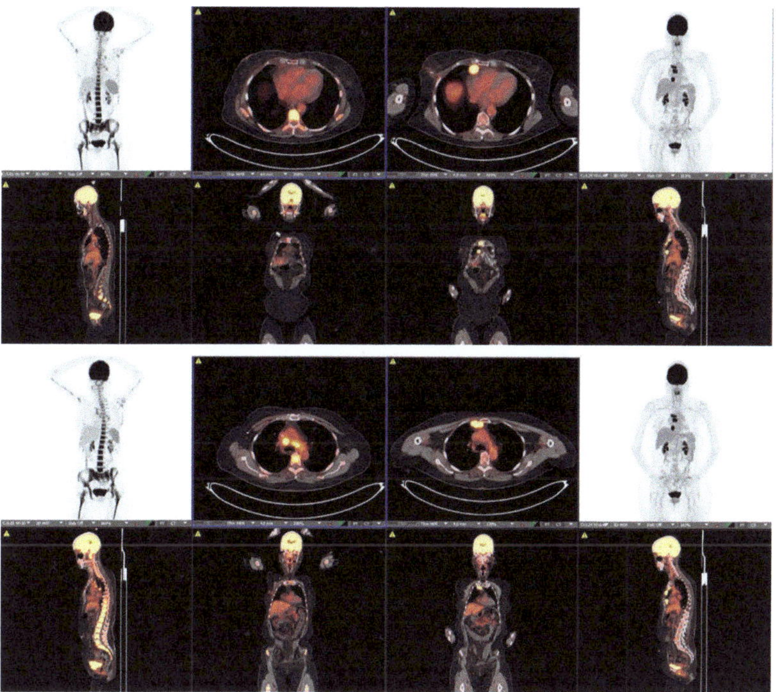

C. Y. O. Wong, D. Wu, *Phenotypic Oncology PET*,
https://doi.org/10.1007/978-3-031-09737-9_27

27.1   Case 27: Interpretation and Teaching

A1:   F-18 FDG.

A2:   No progression. There is new avid uptake at the mediastinal and left hilar (2R, 4R, 7, and 10L) nodes with SUV 8.02 which is likely reactive from immunotherapy.

A3:   The prior hypermetabolic right internal mammary and right pericardiophrenic adenopathy compatible with metastasis has responded drastically well after chemo-immunotherapy.

Reference (*cf* = compared to last PET): Background mediastinal blood pool activity has SUV maximum of 2.58 cf 2.70, and background hepatic parenchymal activity has SUV maximum of 3.29 cf 3.81.

Postsurgical changes are present in the right breast and axilla related to lumpectomy and sentinel lymph node resection. No abnormal radiotracer uptake is present in these operative beds to suggest local tumor recurrence. No hypermetabolic lesion or mass is present in either breast. No avid axillary adenopathy.

There is marked reduction of several enlarged and intensely hypermetabolic right internal mammary lymph nodes from metastatic tumors. The prior most superior lesion is a bilobed nodal conglomerate measuring 10 × 30 mm with SUV maximum of 14.22 (lower image), and another large right internal mammary node extruding into the intercostal space and slightly compressing the pleura measuring 16 × 17 mm with SUV maximum of 17.28 has reduced to SUV 2.51 (left panel). There is no new focal activity on the right lateral aspect of the sternum. The large right pericardiophrenic 17 × 26 mm node with SUV maximum of 17.64 (right sagittal images) is also reduced to 14 × 5 mm with SUV 2.19.

Teaching Point There is new avid uptake at the mediastinal and left hilar nodes which is likely reactive from immunotherapy in view of regression of prior known avid metastasis.

Reference

Gandy N, Arshad MA, Kathryn L, Wallitt K, et al. Immunotherapy-related adverse effects on ^{18}F-FDG PET/CT imaging. Br J Radiol. 2020;93:20190832.

Chapter 28
Case 28: Squamous Cell Lung Cancer

A: This is a 76-year-old female with right lung cancer by CT-guided biopsy showing invasive squamous cell carcinoma (SCC) for initial staging. (1) What is the tracer? (2) Is uptake at right upper lobe metastasis or synchronous or second primary tumor? (3) What other investigation is suggested for differentiation?

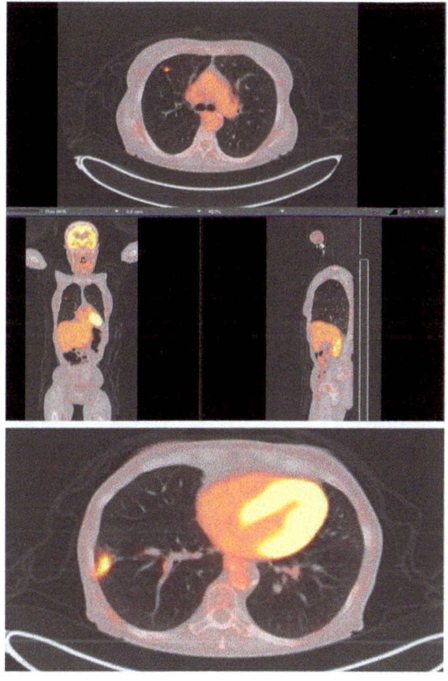

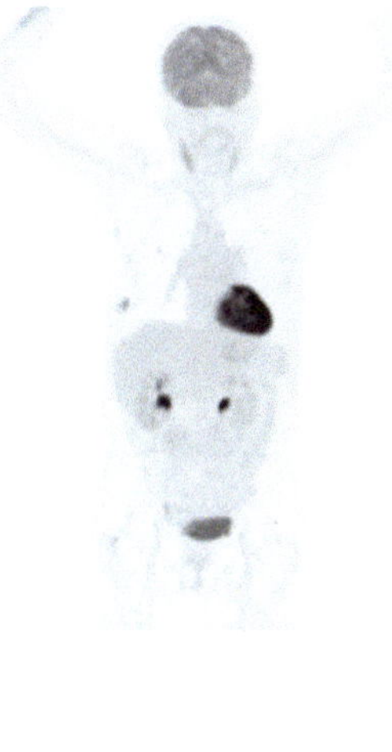

C. Y. O. Wong, D. Wu, *Phenotypic Oncology PET*,
https://doi.org/10.1007/978-3-031-09737-9_28

28.1 Case 28: Interpretation and Teaching

A1: F-18 FDG.

A2: The spiculated nodule 2.8 × 1.1 cm at the lateral aspect of the right lower lobe is avid SUV 4.85 which is biopsied to be SCC. Another 4 mm tiny nodule is noted at the right anterior upper lobe (SUV 3.06) that is suspicious of malignancy though inflammation is also possible. If it is malignant, it may represent a synchronous SCC or metastasis with second primary less likely. There are no abnormal focal areas of increased uptake in the rest of lungs.

A3: If tissue confirmation or clonal assay is not available, further imaging monitor will be helpful. Since pretreatment PET/CT scan, 5-month follow up CT chest post-SBRT showed the biopsy-proven malignancy right lower lung to be less confluent, although its overall size is at 2.2 × 1.4 cm (images not shown). There is greater confluence of the mass density involving the right upper lung anteriorly that measures 2.1 × 0.7 cm for which malignancy is suspected. Interval development elongated 25.5 × 6.1 mm nodule left upper lung is likely inflammatory while CT brain, abdomen and pelvis remains negative.

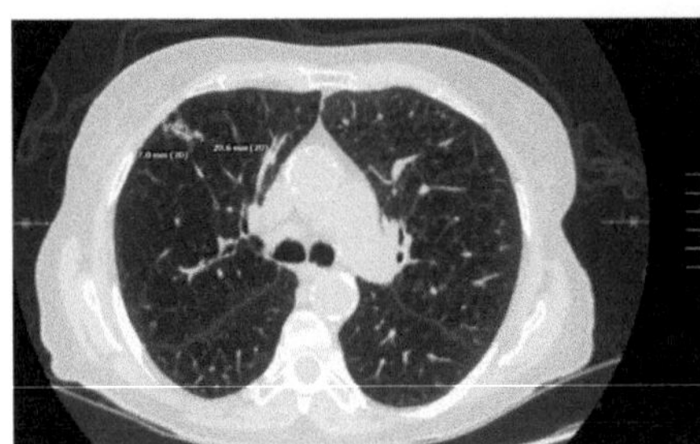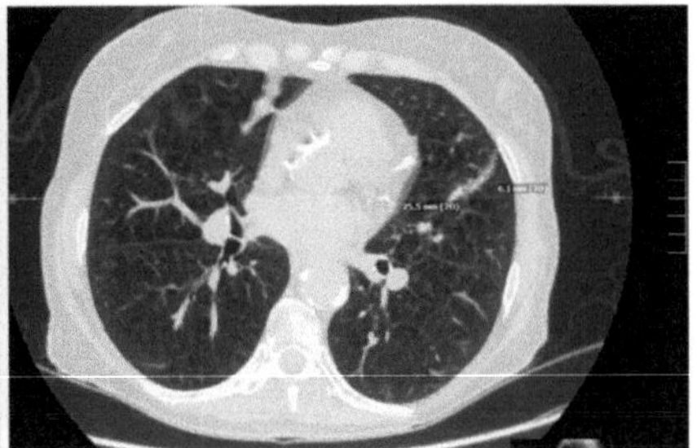

Teaching Point Most common cause of lung nodule in the patient with non-lung cancer is metastasis (over 60%). Multiple pulmonary nodules (>5 mm) and cavitation are the two characteristics associated with the highest chances of metastatic disease. However, squamous cell lung cancer has a small chance of synchronous squamous cell cancer lesion in about 3% of cases instead of metastasis. There is also possible second different primary lung cancer. Thus, the clonal analysis of the lesions is essential.

Reference

Caparica R, Mak MP, Rocha CH, et al. Pulmonary nodules in patients with non-pulmonary cancer: not always metastases. J Global Oncol. 2016;3:138–44.

Chapter 29
Case 29: Lymphoma and Breast Cancer

A: This is a 74-year-old female with diffuse large B-cell (DLBC) lymphoma (from lymph node, right neck biopsy: EBV+) (right two-column panels from the neck to pelvis) receiving R-CHOP × 3 with intrathecal methotrexate (left two-column panel in corresponding levels) for restaging. (1) What is the tracer? (2) What is Lugano response in nodal areas? (3) Is right breast avid focus a lymphoma or breast cancer?

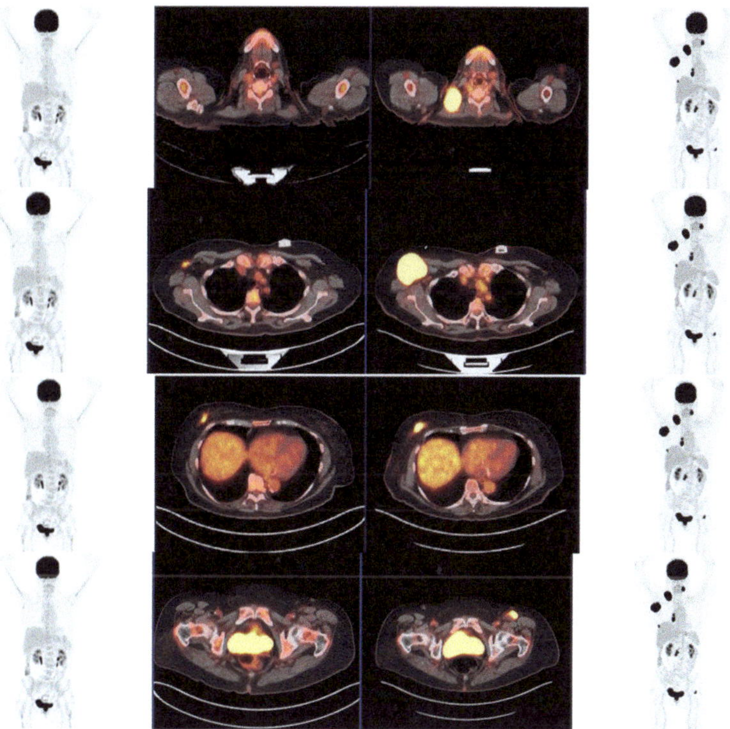

C. Y. O. Wong, D. Wu, *Phenotypic Oncology PET*,
https://doi.org/10.1007/978-3-031-09737-9_29

29.1 Case 29: Interpretation and Teaching

A1: F-18 FDG.

A2: Lugano criteria 2 because there are no residual nodes higher than that of liver except for the right axillary node. The details are provided as below.

The prior 52 × 33 mm right level 5/supraclavicular node with SUV 49.7 is reduced to SUV 2.22 measuring 9 × 3 mm. The prior 25 × 20 mm left level 2 lymph node medial to left sternocleidomastoid muscle with SUV 47.3 has resolved. The prior bulky right axillary nodal mass measuring 56 × 50 mm in the axial plane with SUV 49.7 has reduced to SUV 3.59 at around 6 × 5 mm with metallic clips. The prior 12 × 9 mm medial right subpectoral node with SUV 2.4 has resolved. The prior avid lymphadenopathy in right pulmonary hilar region with SUV 45.3 has reduced to background SUV 2.69. The prior 35 × 21 mm soft tissue density within superior right psoas musculature which demonstrates SUV 38.3 has reduced to SUV 2.96 at around 15 × 7 mm. The prior soft tissue density anterior superior left thigh subcutaneous soft tissues abutting quadriceps musculature measuring 36 × 12 mm in the axial plane with SUV 19.6 has resolved.

Reference SUV (cf = compared to prior PET): SUV in mediastinal blood pool is 2.27 (cf 2.83) and liver is 3.49 (cf 3.63). Lugano response criteria 2 in all nodal areas (excellent response) except in the possible right breast cancer axillary drainage node 3X.

A3: The prior soft tissue mass within right breast glandular tissue measuring 28 × 18 mm with SUV 14.1 has reduced to SUV 4.74.

Although the initial metabolic phenotype in right axilla showed typical DLBC lymphoma as in the recent biopsy, the initial metabolic phenotype in right breast (with lower SUV than the rest of nodes) suggested a possible separate breast cancer.

Recent tissue diagnosis:

1. Lymph node, right axilla, biopsy:

   (a) Diffuse large B-cell lymphoma, germinal center immunophenotype.

2. Right breast, 6, 4 cm from nipple, ultrasound-guided core biopsy:

   (b) Invasive mammary carcinoma with cribriform pattern.

Teaching Point There has been discrepancy between FDG uptake in nodal areas and right breast suggesting likely two different primary malignancies which have discordant uptake before and after treatment. High-grade lymphoma showed significantly higher uptake than lymphoma of lower grade.

Reference

Wong CYO, Thie J, Parling-Lynch KJ, Zakalik D, et al. Glucose-normalized standard uptake value (suv) from f-18 fdg pet in classifying lymphomas. J Nucl Med. 2005;46(10):1659–63.

Chapter 30
Case 30: Prostate Cancer

A: Castration-resistant prostate cancer (27.1 cc T2A, Gleason score = 3 + 3 = 6) post-focal cryoablation therapy at right apex and ADT (androgen deprivation therapy) 3 years ago. PSA is 1.16 (normal 0–4.0 ng/ml) and testosterone is 20 (normal 240–871 mg/dl) when current PET is done (left two-column panel). PSA and testosterone level are 0.65 and 24 (while on ADT), 0.46 and 16 (on ADT), 5.93 and 16 (on ADT when initial PET was done, right panel with yellow exclamation mark), and 0.39 (on ADT), respectively, about 1 month, 1 year, 3 years, and 5 years ago. Recent biopsy showed Gleason 4 + 3 = 7 at left apex and 3 + 3 = 6 at left mid gland based on MRI. The baseline testosterone was 345 about 9 years ago before ADT and PSA was 13 (not on ADT; post-cryoablation) 3 years ago. (1) What are the tracers? (2) Is uptake at prostate gland abnormal in the initial PET (right panel)? (3) Is the ADT effective? (4) There is uptake at left inguinal region in the initial PET (right panel on MIP). What is the likely etiology? (5) Is there evidence of metastasis? Is the bone scan useful for bone metastasis?

C. Y. O. Wong, D. Wu, *Phenotypic Oncology PET*, https://doi.org/10.1007/978-3-031-09737-9_30

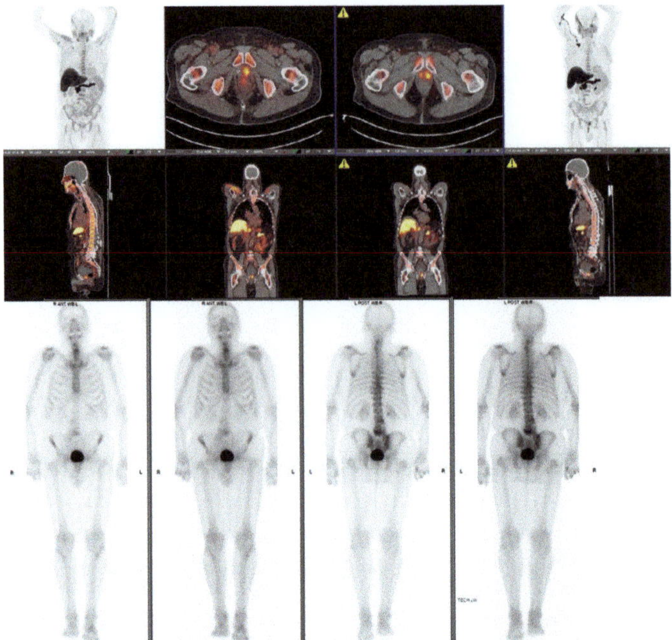

30.1   Case 30: Interpretation and Teaching

A1:   F-18 fluciclovine.

A2 and A3:   Reference (cf=compared to baseline PET): The 1. cm blood pool mean SUV is 1.26 cf 1.47 and the 1.5 cm L3 marrow mean SUV is 4.34 cf 4.98. There is focally increased uptake in the residual prostate gland, post-cryoablation with a persistent area of increased uptake in the slightly larger left lobe (SUV 5.19 cf 11.01) compared to the right (SUV 3.13 cf 5.78). This persistently increased uptake in the left side of prostate gland is consistent with residual or recurrent tumor. The ADT is effective as SUV on both sides have reduced.

A4:   The prior focus of increased uptake (SUV 6.35) in an approximately $12 \times 10 \times 17$ mm left inguinal node has resolved likely inflammatory.

A5:   There is normal diffuse increased uptake in the bone marrow of the axial and appendicular skeleton. There is no avid uptake in the left and right inguinal or iliac nodes or elsewhere. There is no evidence of metastasis. Bone scan is not useful as PSA needs to be over 8 before it can show metastasis.

The initial PET showed evidence of tumor sites on the left side gland based on MRI findings (T2 size $1.4 \times 0.6 \times 0.9$ cm at the left apex and $0.9 \times 0.9 \times 0.7$ cm at left mid gland) consistent with recent biopsy results.

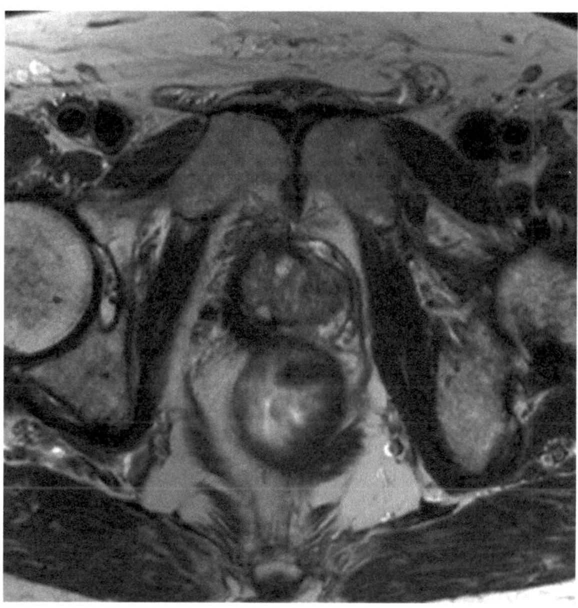

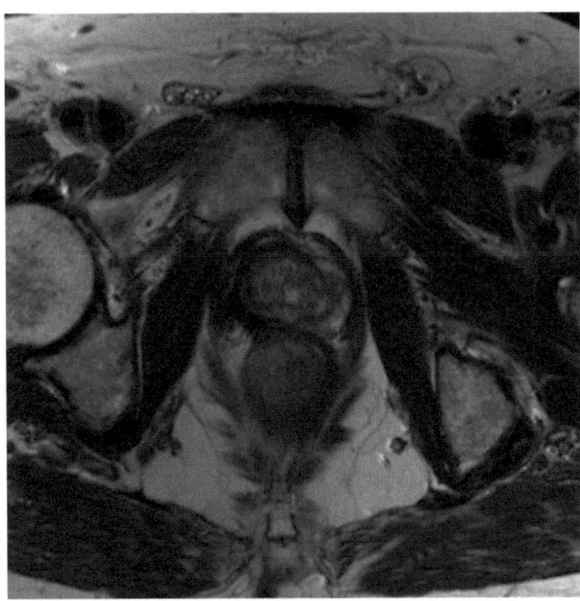

Teaching Point In modern ADT, the PSA level may be very low and metastatic work-up by bone scan is insensitive. The prostate-specific PET agent such as PSMA or fluciclovine is indicated when there is rising PSA.

Reference

Freitas JE, Gilvydas R, Ferry JD, Gonzalez JA. The clinical utility of prostate-specific antigen and bone scintigraphy in prostate cancer follow-up. J Nucl Med. 1991;32(7):1387–90.

Chapter 31
Case 31: Neurofibromatosis and Cerebellar Encephalomalacia

A: PET-CT was performed on a 51-year-old female with history of neurofibromatosis, hydrocephalus status post-VP shunt placement. (1) What is the tracer? (2) What is the diagnosis on the left cerebellum? (3) What are other findings in the body?

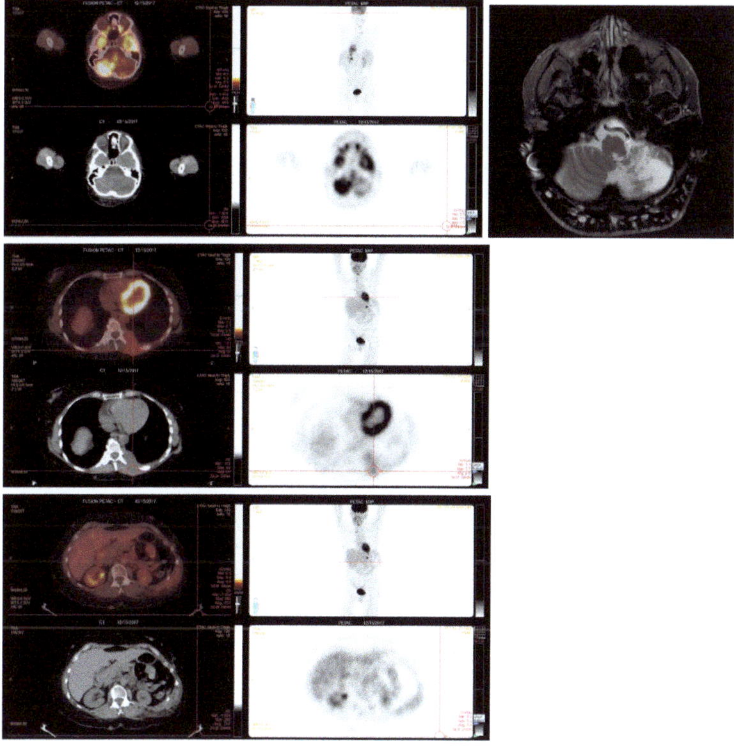

C. Y. O. Wong, D. Wu, *Phenotypic Oncology PET*,
https://doi.org/10.1007/978-3-031-09737-9_31

31.1   Case 31: Interpretation and Teaching

A1:   F-18 FDG.

A2:   Left cerebellar hypometabolism is noted, in line with encephalomalacia on MR imaging, likely due to neuroma mass effects or infarct or both.

A3:   Body images show neuromas in variable sizes, from left para-spinal/pleural mass extending into the left posterior chest wall to tiny cutaneous or subcutaneous nodules, with no appreciable or mild FDG activities, max SUV 3.7. Innumerous cutaneous and subcutaneous nodules are noted in the concurrent CT and the MR imaging.

Teaching Point Neurofibromatosis is characterized by numerous cutaneous and subcutaneous nodules in the peripheral and the central nervous system, with no appreciable or mild FDG activity on PET imaging. Due to high background FDG activity, it's imperative to scale down the FDG activity in the brain when reviewing any appreciable focal abnormality as shown in this case. High uptake at the nodular lesion suggests malignant peripheral nerve sheath tumors (MPNST).

Reference

Meany H, Dombi E, James Reynolds J, et al. 18-fluorodeoxyglucose-positron emission tomography (fdg-pet) evaluation of nodular lesions in patients with neurofibromatosis type 1 and plexiform neurofibromas (PN) or malignant peripheral nerve sheath tumors (MPNST). Pediatr Blood Cancer. 2013;60(1):59–64.

Chapter 32
Case 32: Mucinous Colonic Adenocarcinoma

A: A 76-year-old male undergoing a restaging PET-CT 3 weeks post-right hemico-lectomy due to mucinous colonic adenocarcinoma. (1) What is the tracer? (2) What is the diagnosis of small non-avid node and mesenteric nodules?

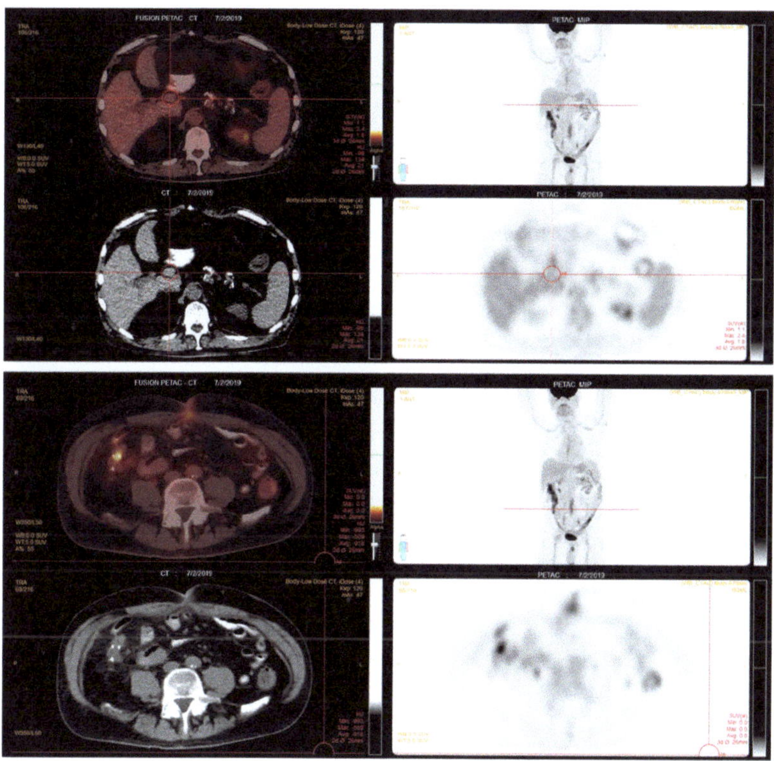

C. Y. O. Wong, D. Wu, *Phenotypic Oncology PET*,
https://doi.org/10.1007/978-3-031-09737-9_32

32.1   Case 32: Interpretation and Teaching

A1:   F-18 FDG.

A2:   There is an approximately 1.5 cm precaval node (upper panel), with minimal FDG activity. Multiple small or tiny mesenteric nodules are noted (lower panel), all without appreciable FDG activity.

Three follow-up PET-CTs show steady progression of omental/peritoneal metastases on left side, suspicious for carcinomatosis, despite chemotherapy and immunotherapy as seen on PET images over 1-year period.

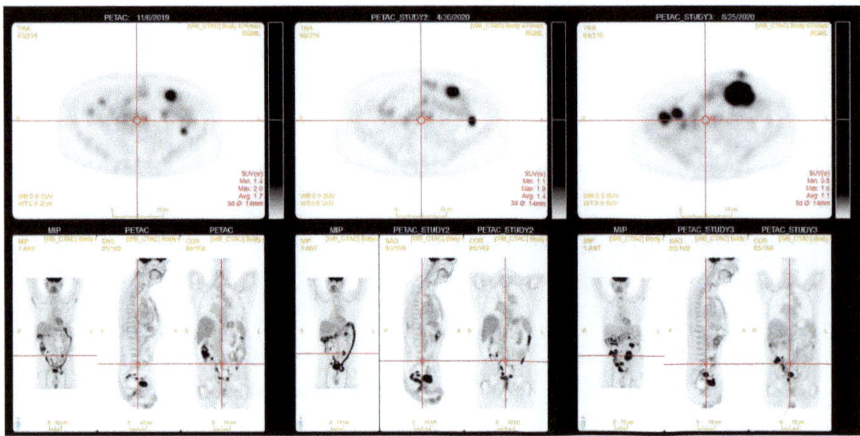

Teaching Point Mucinous adenocarcinomas often have minimal or no appreciable FDG activity, leading to "false-negative" PET study in over 40% of the cases. In fact, this is the feature of low metabolic phenotype. There was a positive correlation between tumor FDG uptake and cellularity but a negative correlation with the amount of mucin. It's imperative to review the CT imaging very carefully as any growing lesions are suspicious of metastases irrespective of low or no uptake on PET. Mucinous adenocarcinomas are often associated with a poor prognosis, as shown in this case.

Reference

Berger KL, Nicholson SA, Dehdashti F, Siegel BA. FDG PET evaluation of mucinous neoplasms: correlation of FDG uptake with histopathologic features. Am J Roentgenol. 2000;174:1005–8.

Chapter 33
Case 33: Poorly Differentiated Gastric Cancer with Signet-Ring Cell Features

A: Initial staging PET-CT in an 80-year-old male with newly diagnosed poorly differentiated gastric adenocarcinoma with signet-ring cell features, via a biopsy of gastric lesser curvature mass 7 days ago. (1) What is the tracer? (2) What are the staging and prognosis?

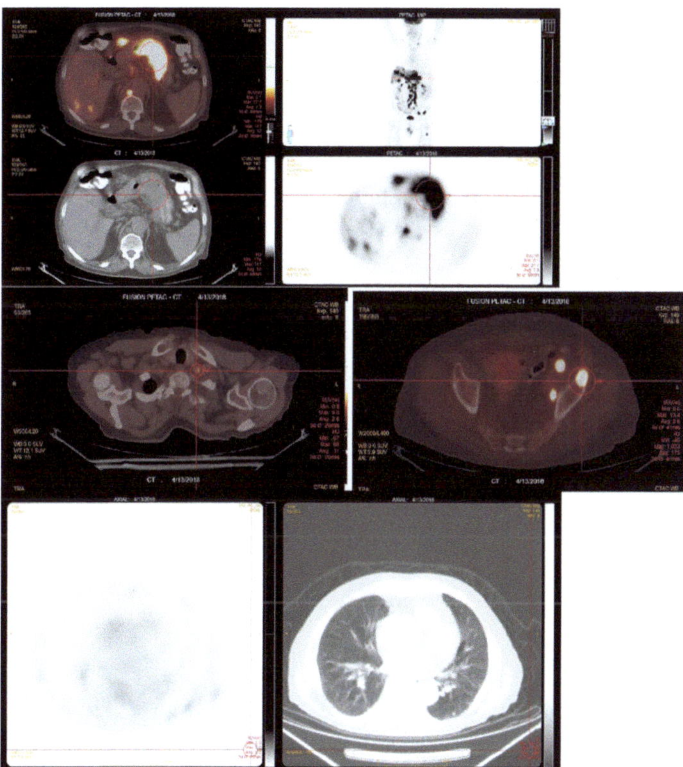

C. Y. O. Wong, D. Wu, *Phenotypic Oncology PET*,
https://doi.org/10.1007/978-3-031-09737-9_33

33.1   Case 33: Interpretation and Teaching

A1:   F-18 FDG.

A2:   Stage IV gastric cancer. PET-CT shows diffuse gastric wall thickening with abnormal FDG activity, max SUV 27.7 (upper panel), as well as numerous paragastric nodal, bilateral retrocrural, and multiple intrahepatic metastases. There is a left supraclavicular prominent node with moderate FDG activity, max SUV 9.0 (middle left), consistent with classical Virchow's nodal metastasis together with other abdominal-pelvic nodes (projection image). Review of lung window imaging (lower panel) two small pulmonary nodules in the lateral posterior subpleural left lower lobe, both without appreciable FDG activity on PET, and at least two similar small nodules in right upper lobe (not shown), suspicious for bilateral lung metastases with a low metabolic rate. Numerous FDG-avid lytic bone lesions (middle row right image), suspicious for multiple bone/bone marrow metastases.

Teaching Point Mucinous gastric adenocarcinoma with signet-ring cell features is a highly aggressive malignancy, often presenting with extensive metastases at the initial diagnosis, with an extremely poor prognosis. SUV are important in estimating prognosis and follow-up of patients. Significant correlation is observed between SUV and the primary size of tumors. The gastric cancers with high FDG uptake tend to have higher malignant aggressiveness as there is significant correlation between the primary tumor SUV and lymph node metastases. Indeed, this 80-year-old male patient passed away 10 days after the PET-CT study, due to quickly deteriorating conditions and multi-organ failure.

Reference

Chen J, Cheong JH, Yun MJ, et al. Improvement in preoperative staging of gastric adenocarcinoma with positron emission tomography. Cancer. 2005;103:2383–90.

Chapter 34
Case 34: Granulomatous Disease Involving Lungs, Lymph Nodes, and Multiple Bones

A: Diagnostic and dual-time PET-CT was performed for evaluation of bilateral lung nodules and mediastinal/hilar adenopathy. (1) What is the tracer? (2) What is the diagnosis? (3) What is the next step of investigation?

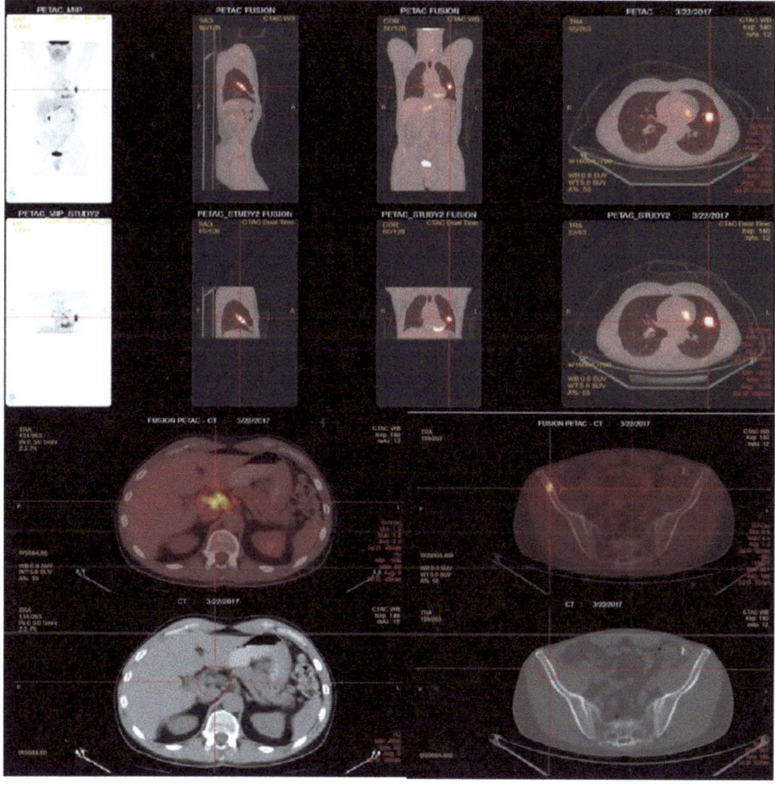

C. Y. O. Wong, D. Wu, *Phenotypic Oncology PET*,
https://doi.org/10.1007/978-3-031-09737-9_34

34.1 Case 34: Interpretation and Teaching

A1: F-18 FDG.

A2: Upper panel confirms the largest lesion in left upper lobe (LUL), with abnormal FDG activity, initial SUV 8.8, increased to 11.7 on delayed PET imaging. Additional bilateral lung nodules show minimal to mild FDG activities, along with FDG-avid bilateral mediastinum and hilar adenopathy. Middle left panel shows FDG adenopathy in the upper abdomen, and middle right panel reveals left anterior iliac crest focal FDG avidity without definite CT correlate for lytic or sclerotic changes. Diagnostic consideration includes metastatic cancer or active sarcoidosis.

A3: Since there is lack of classical pattern of granulomatous disease, tissue sampling is suggested. Biopsy of the dominant FDG-avid LUL lung lesion revealed non-necrotizing granulomatous inflammation, with negative special stains for microorganism. Fourteen months later, a follow-up PET-CT was performed with overall stable findings in comparison to the baseline PET-CT study.

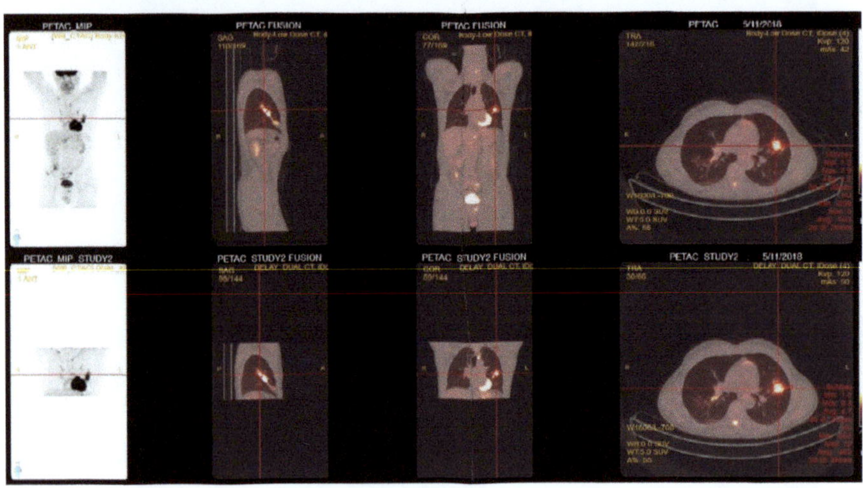

Teaching Point Granulomatous disease is a benign condition that could affect multiple organs/tissues, although the most common sites are the lungs and mediastinum/hila. FDG activity of granulomatous disease could be very variable, as shown in this case, and FDG activity could be increased on delayed PET imaging. The bilateral/symmetric distribution pattern and calcifications in the nodes, above and below diaphragm, in an atypical cancer drainage pattern, liver, or spleen are suggestive of granulomatous disease. Multiple bone involvement without definite CT correlate for lytic or sclerotic changes is also suggestive of granulomas. Clinical and radiographic correlation is highly valuable. If concerns for malignancy/metastasis remain, biopsy of representative lesion for definite diagnosis is recommended.

Reference

Chundru S, Wong CO, Wu D, et al. Granulomatous disease: is it a nuisance or an asset during PET/computed tomography evaluation of lung cancers? Nucl Med Comm. 2008;29(7):623–7.

Chapter 35
Case 35: Lung Nodules in Esophageal Cancer

A: Initial staging PET-CT of biopsy-proven esophageal squamous cell carcinoma via endoscopic biopsy of proximal esophageal mass. (1) What is the tracer? (2) What is the significance of lung nodules? (3) What do you recommend?

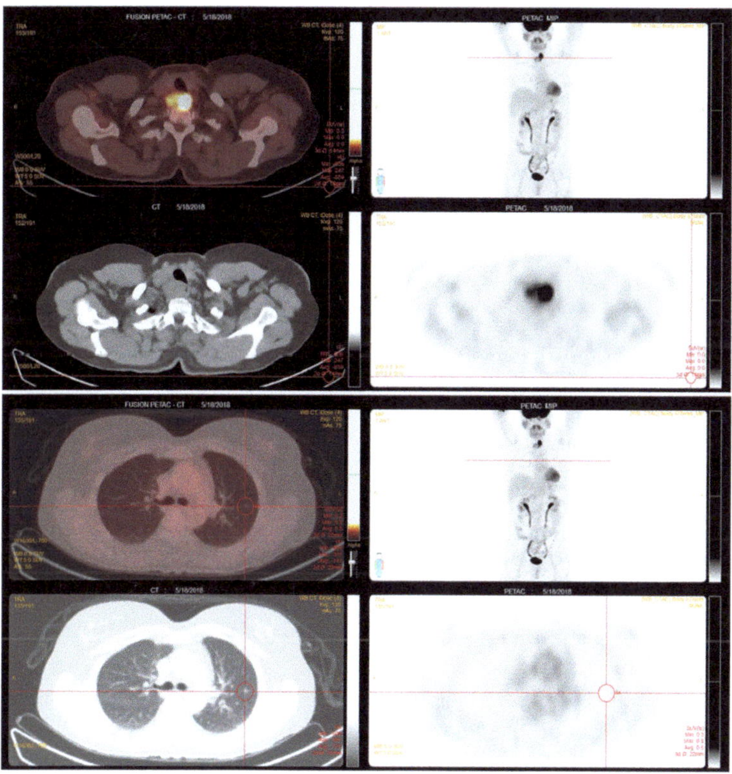

© The Author(s), under exclusive license to Springer Nature Switzerland AG 2022

C. Y. O. Wong, D. Wu, *Phenotypic Oncology PET*,
https://doi.org/10.1007/978-3-031-09737-9_35

35.1 Case 35: Interpretation and Teaching

A1: F-18 FDG.

A2: The staging PET-CT (upper panel) shows proximal esophageal primary malignancy and adjacent adenopathy with a large central necrosis. Multiple bilateral small or tiny lung nodules show no appreciable FDG activity on the PET imaging (lower panel). Differential diagnosis shall include diffuse pulmonary metastases with a very low metabolic rate versus infectious/inflammatory processes.

A3: Short-term PET-CT after treatment is recommended.

The restaging PET-CT following completion of chemoradiation shows improvement or resolution of the esophageal primary and adjacent nodal metastasis. However, multiple lung nodules are enlarged on CT, with interval increased FDG activity on PET, suspicious for progression of pulmonary malignancy or metastases.

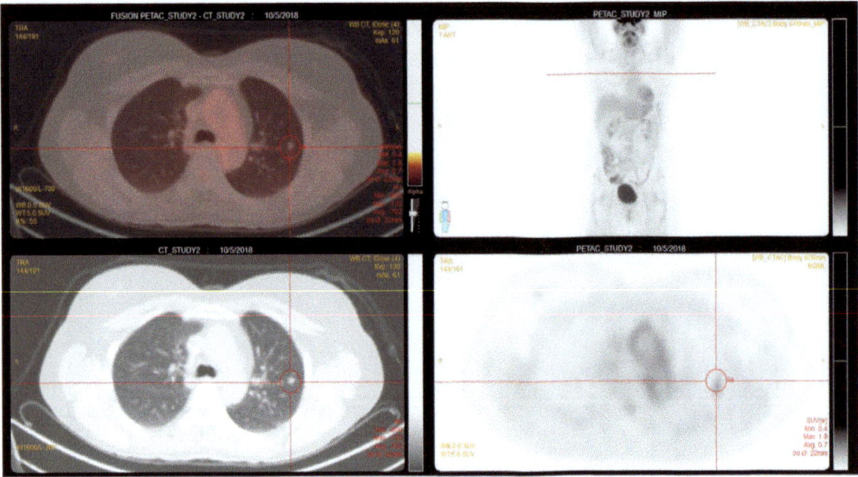

Therefore, the overall PET-CT impression is consistent with a response to recent chemoradiation therapies, with progression of pulmonary metastases or second lung primary tumor.

Teaching Point It's imperative to review CT windows during PET-CT imaging review, and misregistration between CT and PET in lung nodules due to respiratory motion is a common finding. Small size may not be FDG avid due to partial volume effects or low metabolic phenotype. The commonest sites of visceral metastases (M1b) include the lungs, liver, bones, and adrenal glands. Synchronous neoplastic disease can be present in 1.5–5.5% of patients with esophageal cancer at initial presentation.

Reference

Bruzzi JF, Munden RF, Truong MT, et al. PET/CT of esophageal cancer: its role in clinical management. RadioGraphics. 2007;27:1635–52.

Chapter 36
Case 36: Squamous Cell Cancer (SCC) of the Neck

A: Patient is a 94-year-old male with newly diagnosed metastatic SCC of right neck mass via FNA. One week later, PET-CT was performed for initial staging. (1) What is the tracer? (2) What is the primary source of cancer? (3) What is the stage? (4) What is the prognosis?

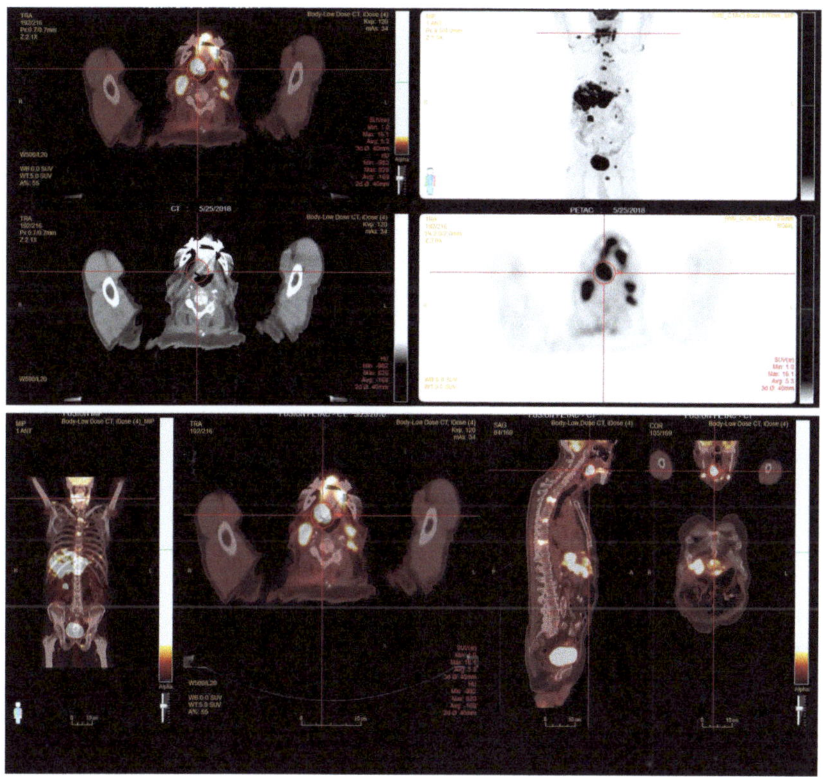

© The Author(s), under exclusive license to Springer Nature Switzerland AG 2022

C. Y. O. Wong, D. Wu, *Phenotypic Oncology PET*,
https://doi.org/10.1007/978-3-031-09737-9_36

36.1 Case 36: Interpretation and Teaching

A1: F-18 FDG.

A2: PET-CT findings are suggestive of right tongue base primary, with max SUV 16.1 (upper panel). Head and neck primary SCC usually skip the posterior cervical nodes except in nasopharyngeal cancer. Lymphoma can involve the posterior and anterior cervical nodes.

A3: Additional findings reveal lymphonodular metastases above and below the diaphragm including bilateral neck, right greater than left, and extensive bone and liver metastasis, which is likely in stage IV (lower panel).

A4: Due to the highly abnormal uptake in PET-CT at multiple sites, the overall prognosis is poor. A core biopsy of liver lesion was performed, with pathology positive for metastatic SCC. Restaging PET-CT was performed to assess treatment response to two cycles of palliative chemotherapy which showed mixed and poor response, with overall progression of metastatic disease (MIP images).

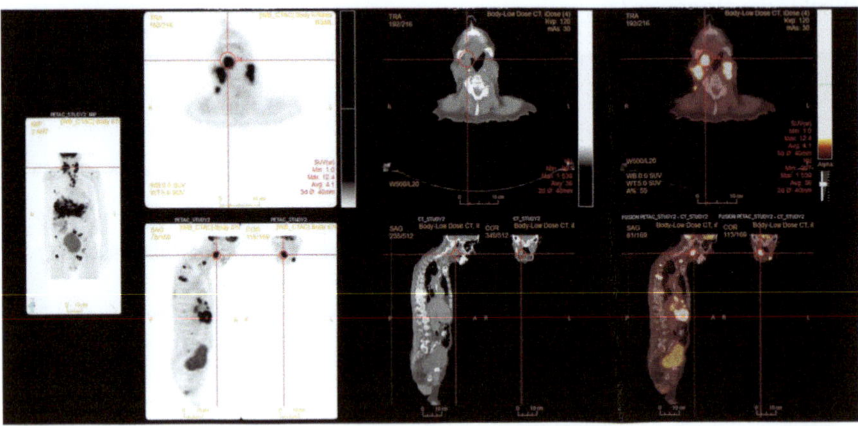

Teaching Point The advanced age, stage IV head/neck cancer, and poor response to chemotherapy are indicating a poor prognosis. Indeed, patient passed away half a year after diagnosis.

Reference

Yoon H, Ha S, Kwon SJ, et al. Prognostic value of tumor metabolic imaging phenotype by FDG PET radiomics in HNSCC. Ann Nucl Med. 2021;35(3):370–7.

Chapter 37
Case 37: Metastatic Prostate Adenocarcinoma

A: Restaging PET-CT in a 57-year-old male with history of castrate-resistant prostate cancer initially receiving multiple treatments including tumor excision, radiation therapy, and multiple lines of chemotherapy currently presents with known extensive metastatic disease involving bones, liver, and retroperitoneal lymph nodes with lower back pain and profound anemia. The most recent PSA level was 1,877.20 ng/ml. (1) What is the tracer? (2) What is the extent of the disease? (3) What is the prognosis?

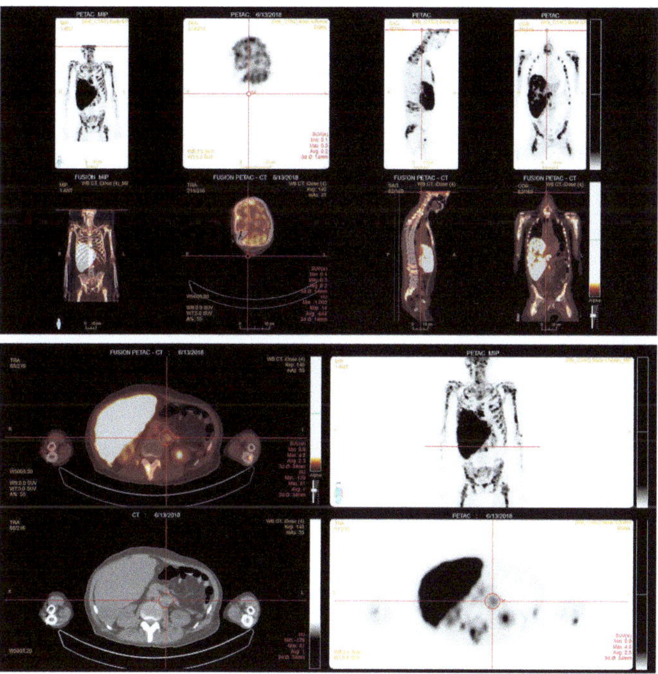

C. Y. O. Wong, D. Wu, *Phenotypic Oncology PET*,
https://doi.org/10.1007/978-3-031-09737-9_37

37.1   Case 37: Interpretation and Teaching

A1:   F-18 FDG.

A2:   PET-CT confirms known metastases involving the skeleton, entire liver, and retroperitoneal lymph nodes. It is an advanced disease.

A3:   The metastatic involvement is extensive and FDG uptake is intense which both indicate a poor prognosis.

Teaching Point FDG PET or PET-CT is not first-line imaging modality for initial staging or restaging of prostate cancers, due to suboptimal sensitivity for detection of primary tumor and metastasis. This leads to the development of new tracers such as F-18 fluciclovine and Ga-68 PSMA. However, FDG PET-CT still has certain value for restaging of advanced metastatic prostate cancer, as shown in case. The extent of metastatic involvement and FDG intensities are two important parameters, along with others, indicating a poor prognosis.

Reference

Shen K, Liu B, Zhou Z, et al. The evolving role of ^{18}F-FDG PET/CT in diagnosis and prognosis prediction in progressive prostate cancer. Front Oncol. 2021, 11:683793.

Chapter 38
Case 38: Mesothelioma

A: Initial PET-CT in a 62-year-old female with newly diagnosed left pleural epithelioid mesothelioma via CT-guided biopsy. (1) What is the tracer? (2) What is the diagnosis?

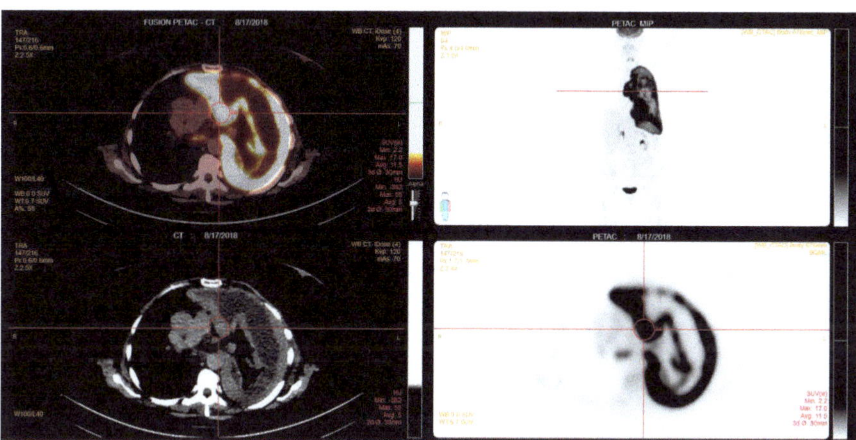

© The Author(s), under exclusive license to Springer Nature
Switzerland AG 2022
C. Y. O. Wong, D. Wu, *Phenotypic Oncology PET*,
https://doi.org/10.1007/978-3-031-09737-9_38

B: Restaging PET-CT after completion of chemotherapy (carboplatin-pembrolizumab-Avastin). (1) What is the response?

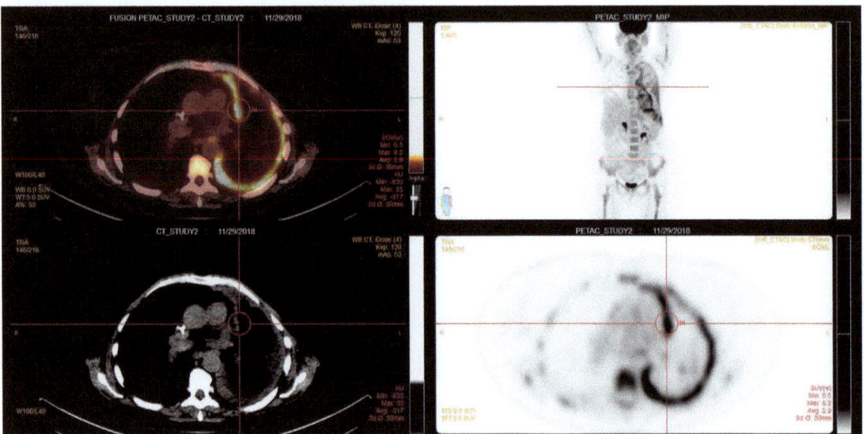

38.1   Case 38: Interpretation and Teaching

A1: F-18 FDG.

A2: Diffuse thickening/nodularity of the entire left parietal and visceral pleura with intense FDG activity suggesting mesothelioma. Lobulated left pleural effusion is present without appreciable FDG activity. Talc pleurodesis may mimic the findings which is often to relieve pleural effusion and its uptake is usually heterogeneous with significant thickening. Pleural biopsy however revealed malignant epithelioid mesothelioma.

B1: The restaging PET-CT shows marked improvement, indicating a favorable but partial response to chemotherapy. The previously noted lobulated pleural effusion has resolved. Diffuse bone marrow uptake is most likely due to reactive changes to recent chemotherapeutic agents.

Teaching Point Generally speaking, stage IV malignant mesothelioma is not surgical candidate. FDG PET-CT plays an important role in the evaluation of systemic treatment response as shown in this case. To get around the problem of false positives with FDG PET-CT in Talc pleurodesis, C-11 choline may be used where inflamed or hardened areas in the pleura do not tend to accumulate C-11 choline intensely.

Reference

Kitajima K, Nakamichi T, Hasegawa S, Kuribayashi K, Yamakado K. Fluorodeoxyglucose versus choline positron emission tomography/computed tomography response evaluation in two malignant pleural mesothelioma patients treated with talc pleurodesis and neoadjuvant chemotherapy. Curcus. 2018;10(11):c3654.

Chapter 39
Case 39: Recurrent Papillary Thyroid Carcinoma

A: Restaging PET-CTs in a 73-year-old male with history of papillary thyroid carcinoma initially diagnosed 2 years ago, status post-total thyroidectomy followed by I-131 therapy/ablation with 158 mCi. The patient also underwent two separate central neck and right lateral neck dissections, both of which yielded metastatic lymph nodes. Unstimulated thyroglobulin was 4.4 ng/ml. (1) What is the tracer? (2) What is the diagnosis?

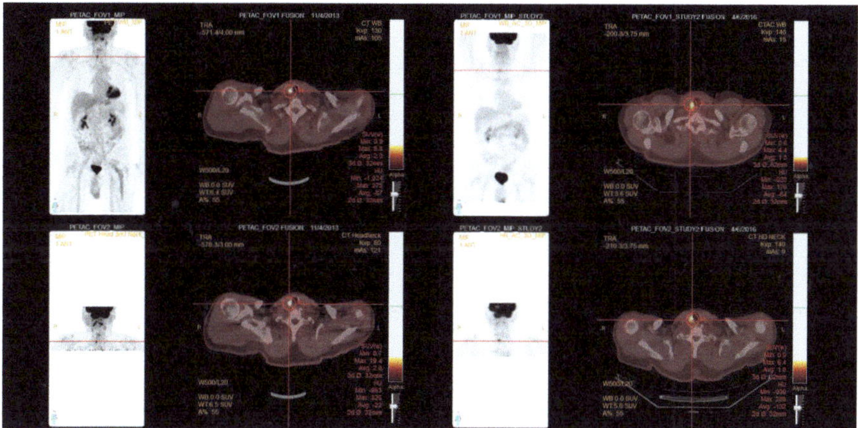

C. Y. O. Wong, D. Wu, *Phenotypic Oncology PET*,
https://doi.org/10.1007/978-3-031-09737-9_39

B: Further PET-CT was performed following FNA positive for anaplastic thyroid carcinoma. (1) What is the tracer? (2) What is the other tracer commonly used for the thyroid cancer? (3) What is the diagnosis?

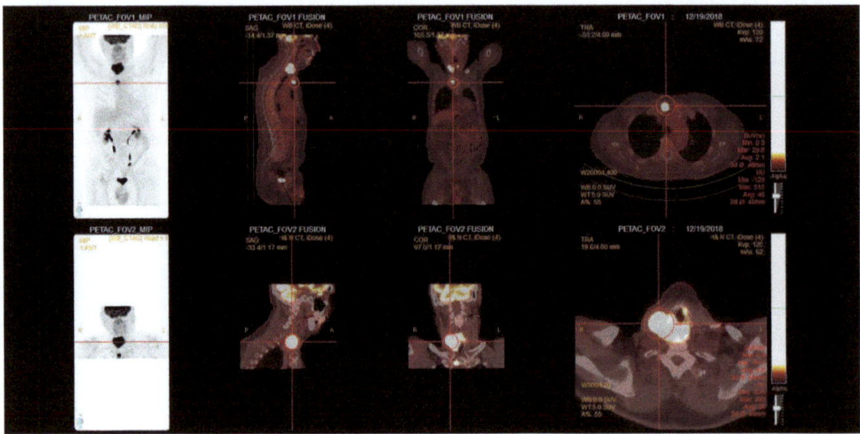

39.1   Case 39: Interpretation and Teaching

A1:   F-18 FDG.

A2:   Recurrent tumor in the right thyroid bed despite repeated neck dissections. Unstimulated thyroglobulin was high and compatible with recurrence.

B1:   F-18 FDG.

B2:   I-131 or I-123 NaI.

B3:   Restaging PET-CT showed right-sided dominant neck mass extending posteriorly crossing the middle line to the left, with intense FDG activity (at least three times higher than the prior study). Also, there is bony metastasis involving the right manubrium. In contrast, I-131 neck and chest whole-body scan is negative.

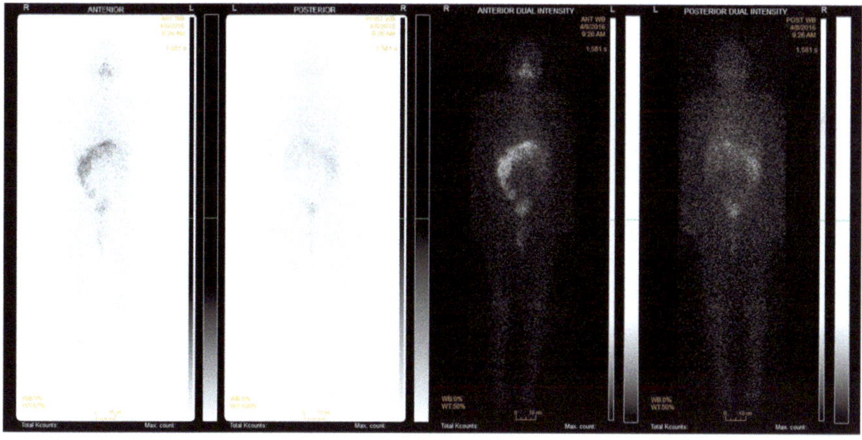

Teaching Point The FDG activity of papillary thyroid cancer and metastasis is often minimal to mild, while anaplastic thyroid cancer is characterized by intense metabolic activity. The discordant finding of FDG PET and I-131 scan, viz., positive FDG but negative I-131 avidity, indicates dedifferentiation of thyroid carcinoma, such as in anaplastic thyroid carcinoma.

Reference

Wong CYO, Dworkin HJ. The role of F-18 FDG PET in metastatic thyroid cancer. J Nucl Med. 1999;40:993–4.

Chapter 40
Case 40: Newly Diagnosed Prostatic Adenocarcinoma

A: Patient is a 70-year-old male with newly diagnosed prostatic adenocarcinoma and Gleason score of 7–8 on the right and 8–9 on the left. PSA level, however, was <0.10 ng/ml. Two months later, PET-CT was performed for initial staging, with measurements as the following with SUV of aorta 2.2 and SUV of L3 vertebral body 4.8. (1) What is the tracer? (2) What are the findings in the prostate? (3) Is there nodal metastasis?

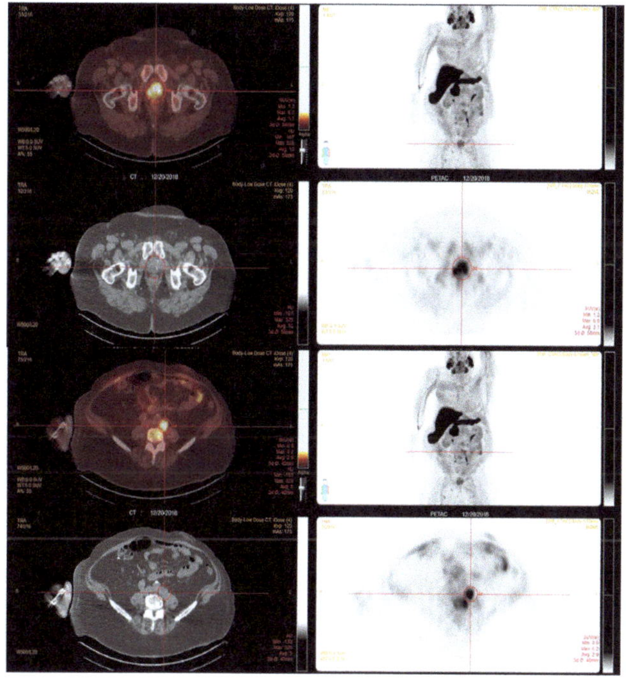

131

C. Y. O. Wong, D. Wu, *Phenotypic Oncology PET*,
https://doi.org/10.1007/978-3-031-09737-9_40

40.1   Case 40: Interpretation and Teaching

A1:   F-18 fluciclovine.

A2:   PET shows mild to moderate tracer activity in both right and left lobes of the prostate, with intensity higher than L3 vertebral body, consistent with biopsy-proven bilobed prostatic carcinoma.

A3:   Yes, there is avid left common aortic node, again with intensity higher than L3 vertebral body; there is another avid mass in the right pelvis (image not shown), which is both suspicious for nodal metastasis.

Teaching Point Mild fluciclovine uptake in prostate gland, especially in the diffuse pattern, is often indicating inflammatory changes. In contrast, moderate fluciclovine uptake with intensity higher than L3 vertebral body is suspicious for or consistent with prostatic primary malignancy or recurrent disease. The prostate cancers detected at lower PSA levels are more likely to have a small volume (less than 0.5 ml).

Reference

Ballentine Carter HB. Prostate cancers in men with low psa levels—must we find them? N Engl J Med. 2004;350(22):2292–4.

Chapter 41
Case 41: Alveolar Rhabdomyosarcoma with a Favorable Response to Chemoradiation

A: Initial staging PET-CT in a 19-year-old male with newly diagnosed right lower extremity alveolar rhabdomyosarcoma, via excisional biopsy of right femoral lymph node. (1) What is the tracer? (2) Where is the primary site of rhabdomyosarcoma? (3) What's the underlying cause of right hydronephrosis?

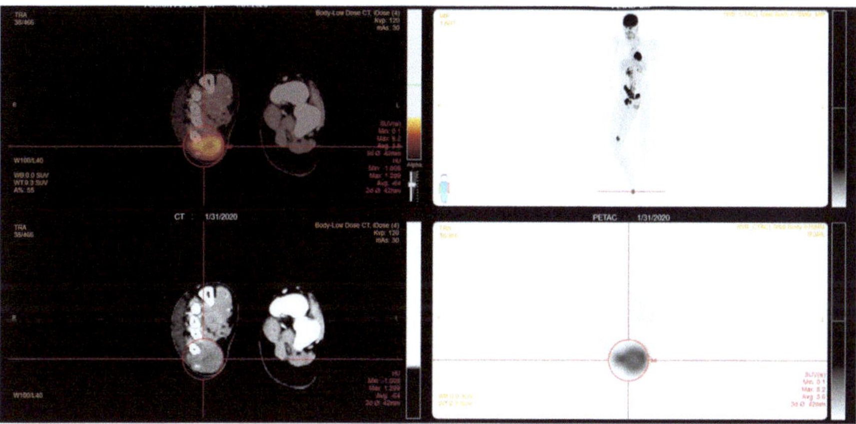

C. Y. O. Wong, D. Wu, *Phenotypic Oncology PET*,
https://doi.org/10.1007/978-3-031-09737-9_41

B: He received chemotherapy and then consolidation radiation therapy to the retroperitoneal and pelvic lymph nodes. Restaging PET-CT scans were performed with images as the following: (1) How was the response to chemotherapy and radiation? (2) What does the mediastinal FDG activity represent in the last two PET? (3) What is the likely cause for the heterogenous FDG activity in the bilateral lower neck at supraclavicular regions? (4) What is the likely cause of the focal FDG activity in the left elbow region?

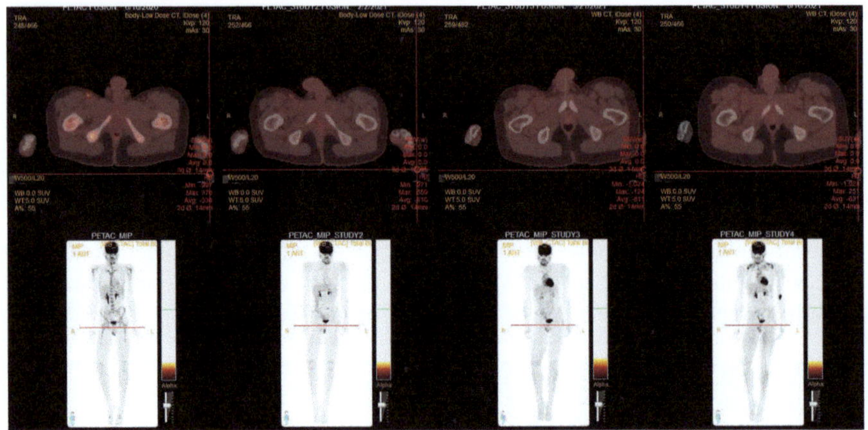

41.1 Case 41: Interpretation and Teaching

A1: F-18 FDG.
A2: Right foot muscle.
A3: Nodal metastasis in the right pelvis.

B1: Excellent response.
B2: Reactive changes to immunotherapy.
B3: Brown fat.
B4: Injection site.

Teaching Point ^{18}F-FDG PET-CT may be useful for patients affected by rhabdo-myosarcoma, in staging, in the evaluation of response to therapy, and for restaging/detection of relapse.

Reference

Donner D, Feraco P, Meneghello L, et al. Usefulness of 18f-FDG PET-CT in staging, restaging, and response assessment in pediatric rhabdomyosarcoma. Diagnostics (Basel). 2020;10(12):1112.

Chapter 42
Case 42: Central Nervous System (CNS) Posttransplant Lymphoproliferative Disorder (PTLD) and Diffuse Large B-Cell Lymphoma (DLBCL)

A: Initial PET-CT in a 60-year-old male with past medical relevant history of renal transplant on chronic immunosuppression, frequent infections including epidural abscess on chronic amoxicillin treatment, and newly diagnosed CNS PTLD/DLBCL, status post-excision of right temporal brain mass. (1) What is the tracer? (2) What is the underlying cause for the diffuse hypometabolism in the right temporal region? (3) Is there any evidence of lymphomatous involvement in the peripheral sites/outside CNS? (4) What does the heterogeneous and moderate FDG activity represent in the right pelvic fossa?

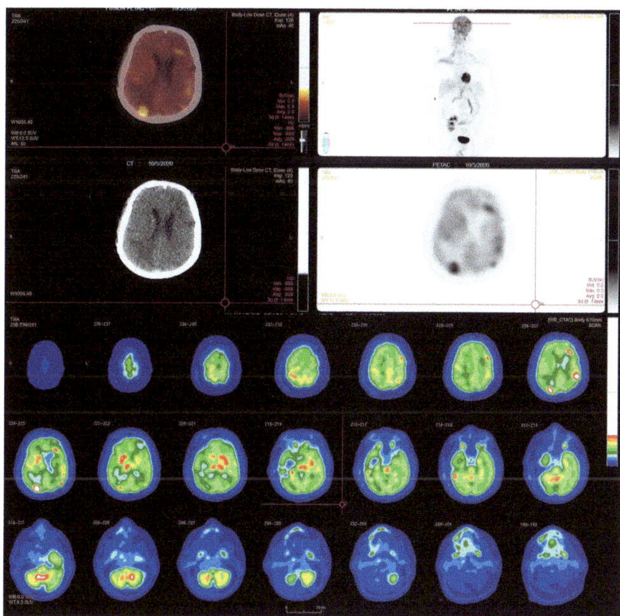

C. Y. O. Wong, D. Wu, *Phenotypic Oncology PET*,
https://doi.org/10.1007/978-3-031-09737-9_42

42.1 Case 42: Interpretation and Teaching

A1: F-18 FDG.

A2: Diffuse right temporal region is likely from secondary diaschisis of the resection. There are other avid foci such as in right parietal and left frontal lobe suggesting multifocal CNS lymphomas.

A3: There is no definite evidence of lymphoma involvement in the peripheral nervous system, although curvilinear FDG activity in the right upper chest wall and in the bilateral accessory respiratory muscles is seen.

A4: Transplant kidney.

Teaching Point The posttransplant lymphoproliferative disorder (PTLD) is a common malignancy after kidney transplant which occurs in 1–3% adult renal transplant recipients and is associated with poor survival rates after diagnosis due to exposure to immunosuppression, impairment of cellular immunity, and the infective agent Epstein-Barr virus (EBV). PTLD tissue is EBV positive in about ¾ of cases. It has a bimodal pattern of incidence, with peaks in the first year and then in the later posttransplantation period. FDG PET often shows intense avidity, suggesting DLBCL as in this case.

Reference

Morton M, Coupes B, Roberts SA, et al. Epidemiology of posttransplantation lymphoproliferative disorder in adult renal transplant recipients. Transplantation. 2013;95(3):470–8.

Chapter 43
Case 43: Solitary Plasmacytoma

A: Initial PET-CT in a 77-year-old male with newly diagnosed plasma cell neoplasm via CT-guided biopsy of left upper retroperitoneal mass 3 months ago. (1) What is the tracer? (2) What does the heterogeneous tracer activity in the left retroperitoneal mass represent? (3) Is there any FDG-avid lesion other than the known malignant mass?

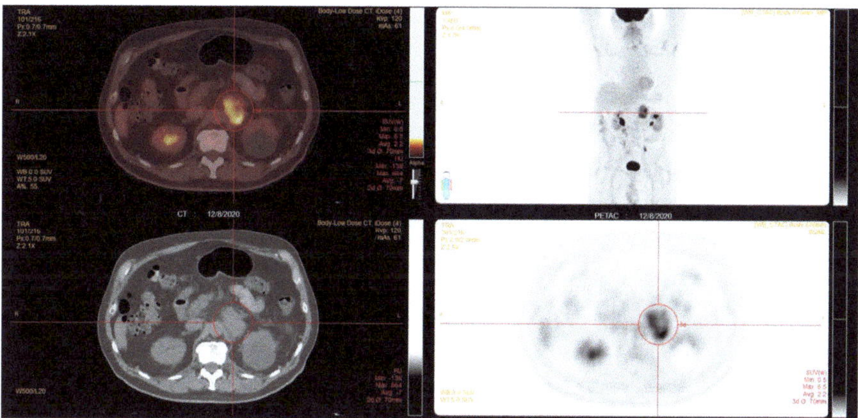

C. Y. O. Wong, D. Wu, *Phenotypic Oncology PET*,
https://doi.org/10.1007/978-3-031-09737-9_43

B: Restaging PET-CT was performed after radiation therapy to the left retroperitoneal plasma cell neoplasm. (1) How was the response to radiation? (2) Is there any new lesion in the right inferior kidney?

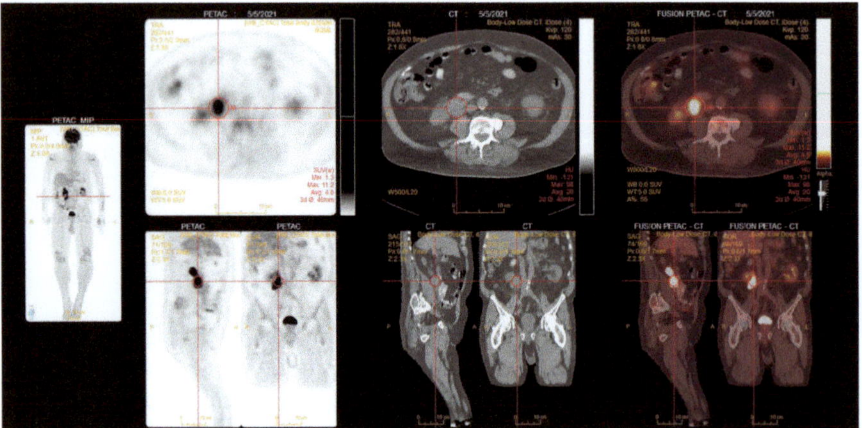

43.1   Case 43: Interpretation and Teaching

A1:   F-18 FDG.
A2:   The heterogeneous tracer activity in the left retroperitoneal mass represents persistent plasma cell neoplasm.

B1:   There is excellent response to local radiation therapy.
B2:   Yes, there is a new lesion in the right inferior kidney.

The patient is put on oral chemotherapy. Bone marrow biopsy was performed twice with half a year apart; both were suspicious for minimally involvement versus reactive changes. A restaging PET-CT was performed.

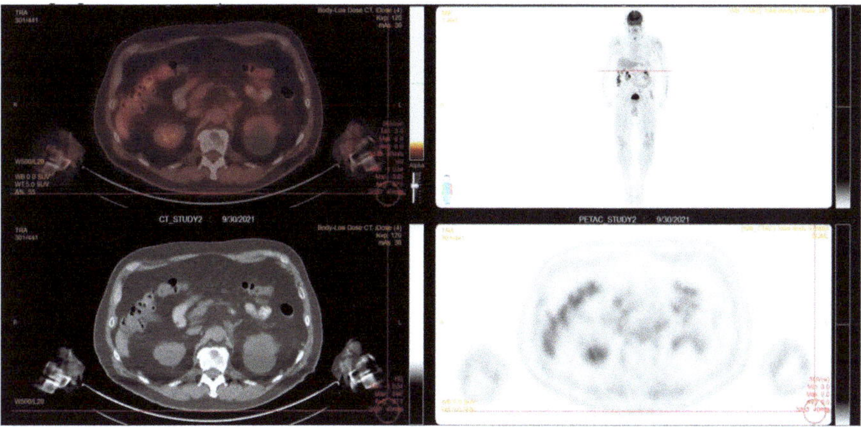

There is excellent response to oral chemotherapy for right renal plasmacytoma. There is photopenic lesion in the kidney, stable since initial PET, likely a left renal cyst.

Teaching Point   Renal plasmacytoma is extremely rare that develops due to uncontrolled plasma cell proliferation and monoclonal plasmacytic infiltration. Extramedullary plasmacytomas are detected in the left retroperitoneal mass which is FDG avid. Renal cysts are hypometabolic.

Reference

Zhang SQ, Dong P, Zhang ZL, et al. Renal plasmacytoma: report of a rare case and review of the literature. Oncol Lett. 2013;5(6):1839–43.

Chapter 44
Case 44: Parotid Oncocytic Carcinoma

A: Initial PET-CT in an 82-year-old male with FNA of left parotid mass showing oncocytic cells and history of prostate cancer. (1) What is the tracer? (2) In addition to FDG-avid left parotid lesion, is there any evidence for lymph node involvement?

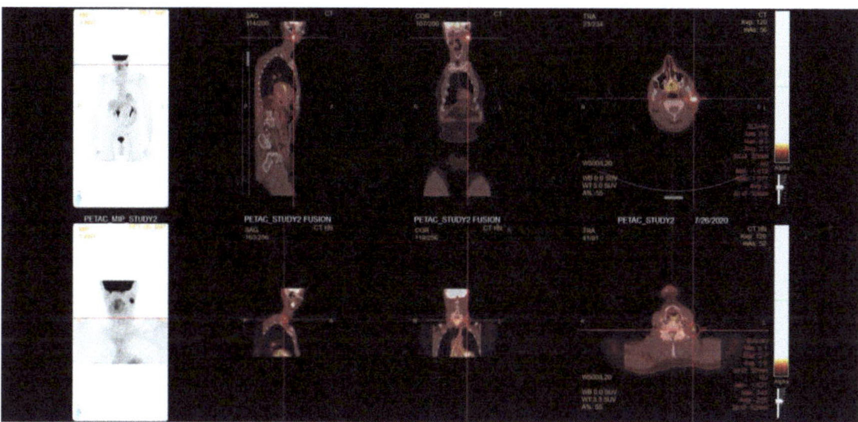

© The Author(s), under exclusive license to Springer Nature Switzerland AG 2022

C. Y. O. Wong, D. Wu, *Phenotypic Oncology PET*, https://doi.org/10.1007/978-3-031-09737-9_44

B: Patient underwent excision of parotid mass and left neck dissection which revealed a main parotid mass and a satellite lesion, both positive for oncocytic carcinoma, and six left neck lymph nodes positive for metastasis. Restaging PET-CT was performed after completion of proton radiation. (1) What is the tracer? (2) How was treatment response? (3) Were the spinal lesions metastasis from parotid primary or prostate primary?

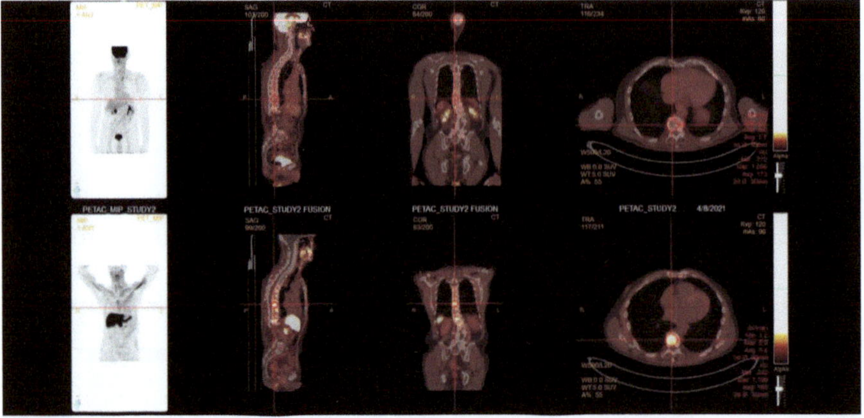

44.1   Case 44: Interpretation and Teaching

A1:   F-18 FDG.
A2:   There is FDG-avid evidence for lymph node involvement.

B1:   F-18 FDG.
B2:   The left parotid neoplasms are treated by precision proton therapy.
B3:   The spinal lesions are avid, mostly likely metastasis from parotid primary rather than prostate primary which is indolent and less avid.

Teaching Point Salivary gland neoplasms may be benign or malignant, and malignant tumors can be primary or metastatic. Most salivary gland tumors occur in the parotid; about 10% occur in the submandibular gland. A good rule of thumb to remember is the rule of 80s in that 80% of all salivary tumors are in the parotid, 80% of parotid tumors are benign, and 80% of the benign tumors that arise in the parotid are pleomorphic adenomas. Warthin's tumor is the second most common benign lesion. Although parotid cancer is rare, it does occur. Approximately 3% of all head and neck neoplasms originate in the parotid gland and less than 1% are oncocytic. Because of the high FDG uptake in some benign tumors, and particularly pleomorphic adenomas, incidental findings in FDG PET need ultrasound scan to further evaluate about the site, size, and nature of salivary gland tumors and the presence of any significant cervical lymphadenopathy. The presence of FDG-avid neck adenopathy is a warning sign of malignancy, as shown in this case.

Patient underwent SBRT to T11, T12, and L3; then a restaging PET-CT was performed.

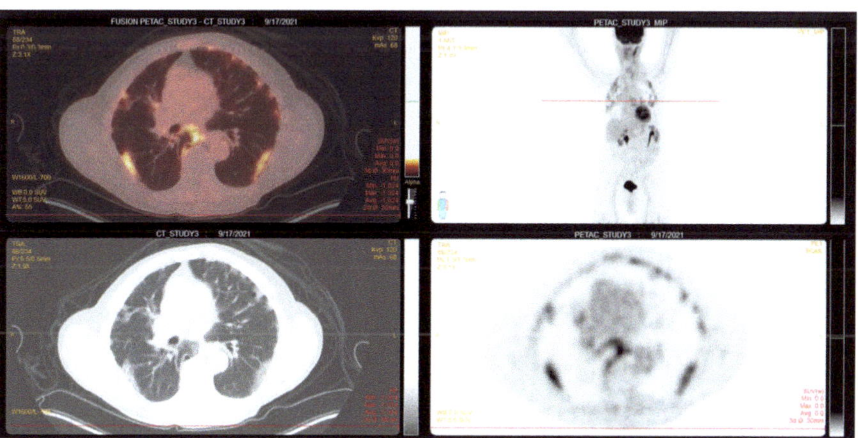

The new lung avid findings are most likely infection or inflammation, recommending COVID-19 test. During the COVID-19 pandemic (referring the date of the imaging in 2021), any newly developed lung opacities, especially in elder patients, shall raise concerns for COVID-19 infection/pneumonia. This patient underwent COVID-19 test for three times, all negative and was followed up clinically.

Reference

Seo YL, Yoon DY, Baek S, et al. Incidental focal FDG uptake in the parotid glands on PET/CT in patients with head and neck malignancy. Eur Radiol. 2015;25(1):171–7.

Chapter 45
Case 45: Pelvis Sarcoma with IVC Metastatic Thrombus

A: Initial staging PET-CT in a 69-year-old female with biopsy-proven right pelvic sarcoma. (1) What is the tracer? (2) What does the large central photopenia within the right pelvic mass represent? (3) What is the likely cause of the lesion within the IVC? (4) What's the nature of the two right upper lobe lung nodules with variable FDG activity?

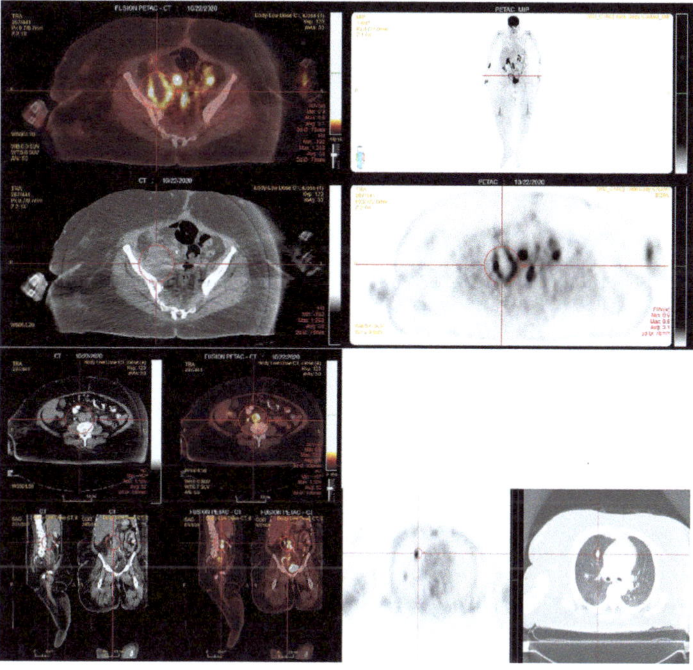

C. Y. O. Wong, D. Wu, *Phenotypic Oncology PET*, https://doi.org/10.1007/978-3-031-09737-9_45

## 45.1	Case 45: Interpretation and Teaching

A1:	F-18 FDG.

A2:	The large central photopenia within the right pelvic mass represents tumor necrosis, which is a typical feature of a sarcoma.

A3:	Tumor embolism is likely the cause of the avid lesion within the IVC.

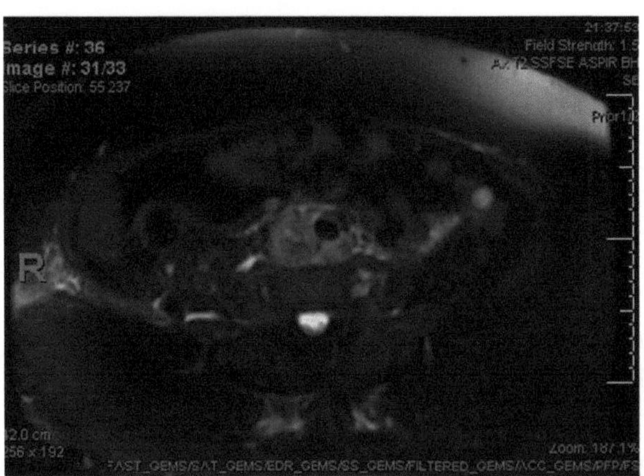

A4:	The nature of the two right upper lobe lung nodules with variable FDG activity is most likely metastasis.

Teaching Point FDG PET-CT can distinguish sarcoma seeding from nonmalignant venous embolism based on the different degree of metabolism with former at least twice as high as the latter which is usually at the level of blood pool activity.

Reference

Ito K, Kubota K, Morooka M, et al. Diagnostic usefulness of 18F-FDG PET/CT in the differentiation of pulmonary artery sarcoma and pulmonary embolism. Ann Nucl Med. 2009;23(7):671–6.

Chapter 46
Case 46: Diffuse Muscle Uptake and Vigorous Exercise

A: Restaging PET-CT in a 66-year-old male with history of invasive moderately differentiated colon cancer treated with right hemicolectomy, completed chemotherapy 3 months ago. The most recent CEA level was 3.1 ng/ml. Patient reported that he ran about 2 miles yesterday, although his blood glucose level was 97 mg/dL at that time of tracer administration. (1) What is the tracer? (2) What's the likely underlying cause for the increased muscle uptake including left ventricular myocardium uptake? What do we recommend?

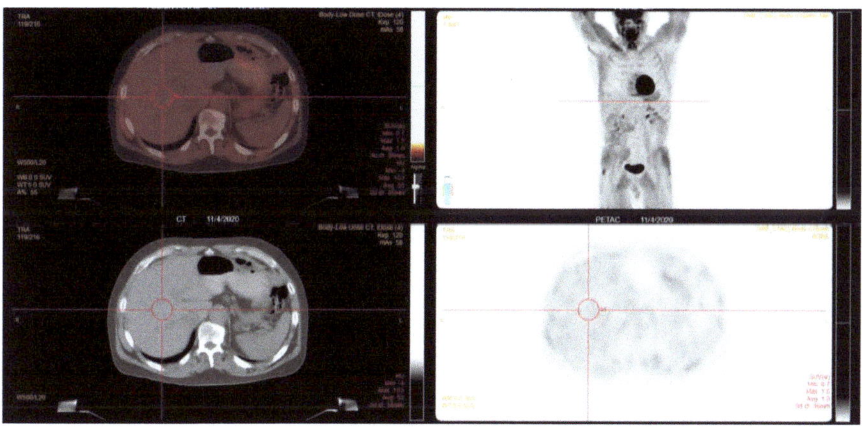

C. Y. O. Wong, D. Wu, *Phenotypic Oncology PET*, https://doi.org/10.1007/978-3-031-09737-9_46

B: After 3.5 months, another restaging PET-CT was performed. The most recent CEA was 2.7 ng/ml. (1) Is the radioactive tracer distribution normal? (2) Is there any evidence of malignancy or metastasis?

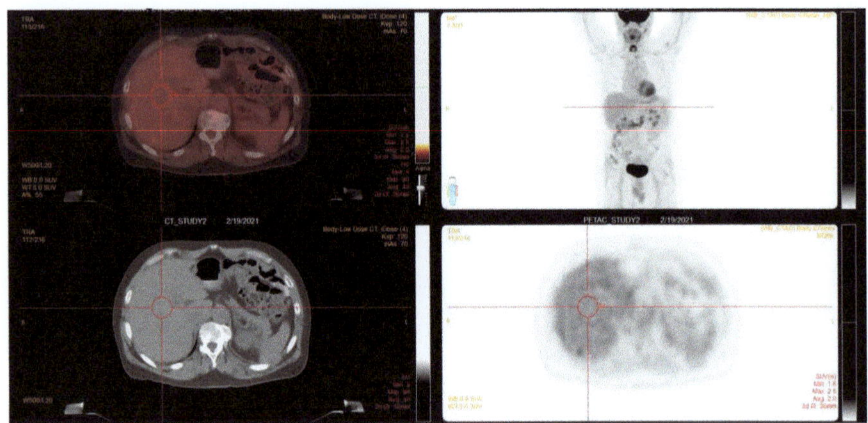

46.1   Case 46: Interpretation and Teaching

A1:   F-18 FDG.
A2:   Vigorous exercise increased muscular uptake from driving force of insulin. Repeat the scan at the resting level after 24 h to reduce recruitment of extra-cardiac muscles with high-carbohydrate diet to reduce cardiac uptake.

B1:   Yes.
B2:   There is a tiny focus of vague uptake at the posterior segment of the liver, suspecting metastasis.

Summarized max SUV between two PET-CT scans

	1st PET-CT (altered distribution)	2nd PET-CT (normal)
Cerebella	6.0	9.8
Mediastinal blood pool	0.7	1.8
versus Lung parenchyma	0.4	0.7
LV myocardium	11.1	5.5
Liver	1.5	2.6
Muscle of right lateral thigh	4.8	2.0

Teaching Point Vigorous exercise such as cross-country run should be avoided at least 48 h prior to appointment for FDG PET-CT study. Once altered FDG distribution is seen, along with diffuse muscle uptake and increased uptake by myocardium, a repeat FDG PET-CT shall be recommended. The standardized protocol recommends that exercises such as jogging, cycling, weight lifting, strenuous housework, and yard work should be avoided for a minimum of 24 h. Patients should also not chew gum for 24 h before the PET scan as this has been shown to activate masticatory muscles.

Reference

Schultz C. The effect of glucose on quality of pet scan results. J of Pharm Pharm. 2017;4(2):138–41. https://doi.org/10.15436/2377-1313.17.018.

Chapter 47
Case 47: Post-excision Residual Urothelial Carcinoma

A: Restaging PET-CT in a 60-year-old male 1 month post-transurethral resection of bladder urothelial carcinoma. Pre-surgical CT image was displayed for comparison: (1) What is the tracer? (2) Does the intense tracer activity represent normal urine activity or residual malignancy? (3) Is there any evidence for peri-bladder invasion?

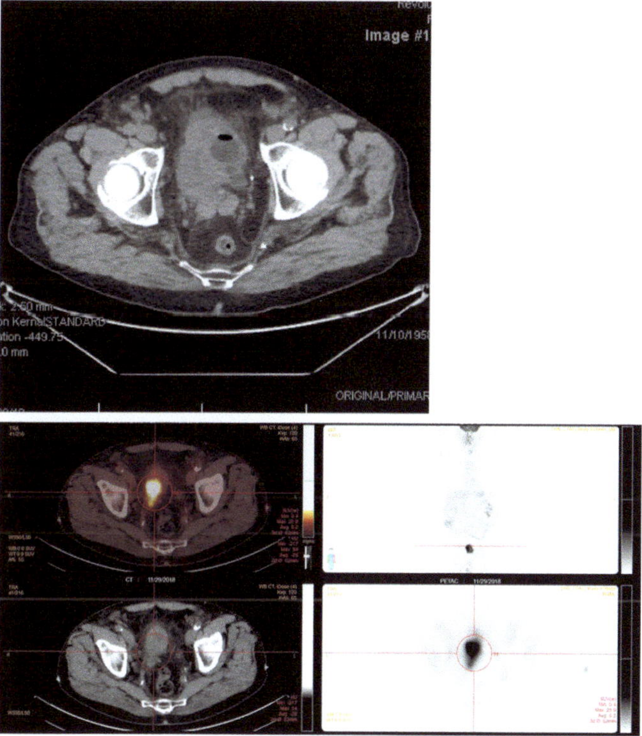

C. Y. O. Wong, D. Wu, *Phenotypic Oncology PET*,
https://doi.org/10.1007/978-3-031-09737-9_47

47.1   Case 47: Interpretation and Teaching

A1:   F-18 FDG.
A2:   The intense tracer activity represents residual malignancy.
A3:   There is evidence for peri-bladder invasion.

Teaching Point Evaluation of bladder urothelial carcinoma is a challenge due to intense normal urine radioactive tracer activity. Scale-down of the intensity is a key to reveal focal abnormal FDG activity other than urine, and correlation with bladder wall thickening or mass-like lesion is imperative to diagnose primary or residual disease. The diagnostic accuracy of FDG PET or PET-CT is good in evaluating metastatic lesions of urinary bladder cancer.

Reference

Lu YY, Chen JH, Liang JA, et al. Clinical value of FDG PET or PET/CT in urinary bladder cancer: a systemic review and meta-analysis. Eur J Radiol. 2012;81(9):211–6.

Chapter 48
Case 48: Phenotypic Pattern
of Erdheim-Chester Disease (ECD)

A: Initial staging PET-CT in a 54-year-old male with newly diagnosed histiocytic neoplasm via biopsy of left thigh/groin mass, with pathologist expert's review suggesting Erdheim-Chester disease (ECD). Medical oncology history is significant for prostate cancer and hemangioblastoma. (1) What is the tracer? (2) In addition to the known left thigh mass, is there any evidence for direct invasion of left femoral head/neck? (3) In the chest, is there any pattern to suggest a benign etiology?

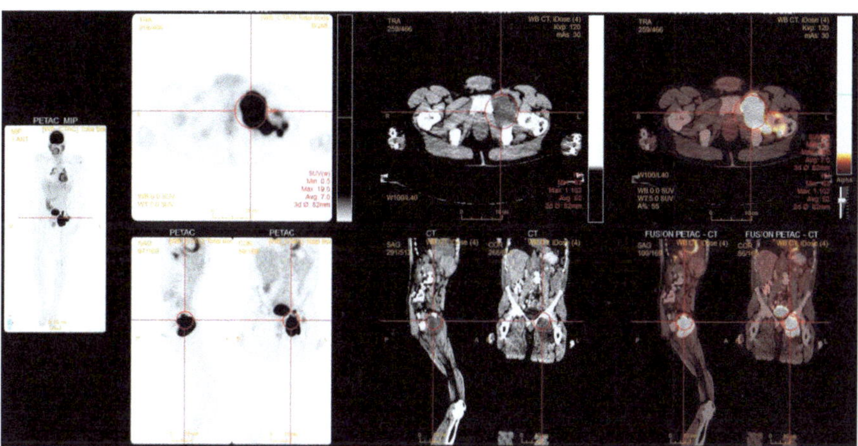

C. Y. O. Wong, D. Wu, *Phenotypic Oncology PET*,
https://doi.org/10.1007/978-3-031-09737-9_48

48.1 Case 48: Interpretation and Teaching

A1:   F-18 FDG.

A2:   Max SUV of the left thigh mass is 19.0, while max SUV of the adjacent left femoral head and neck is 6.0, suspicious for direct invasion.

A3:   Symmetrical hilar distribution suggests a benign etiology from inflammation or granulomatous exposure.

Teaching Point Erdheim-Chester disease (ECD) is a rare multisystem disorder of adulthood, characterized by excessive production and accumulation of histiocytes. The most common sites involved were the skeleton (over 90%), including half with axial and pelvic skeletal involvement, kidneys (over 80%), and central nervous system (CNS) (about 50%). The presence of a BRAF mutation was associated with ^{18}F-FDG-avid CNS disease, the higher SUV_{max}, the greater mortality.

Reference

Young JR, Johnson GB, Murphy RC, et al. (18)F-FDG PET/CT in Erdheim-Chester disease: imaging findings and potential BRAF mutation biomarker. J Nucl Med. 2018;59(5):774–9.

Chapter 49
Case 49: Different Metabolic Phenotypes of Renal Clear Cell Carcinoma and Cervix Cancer

A: Initial staging PET-CT in a 40-year-old female with newly diagnosed renal clear cell carcinoma (RCC) of right kidney and cervix adenocarcinoma. The latter was diagnosed and classified as stage IB. (1) What is the tracer? (2) Are the PET metabolic phenotypes consistent with pathological diagnosis?

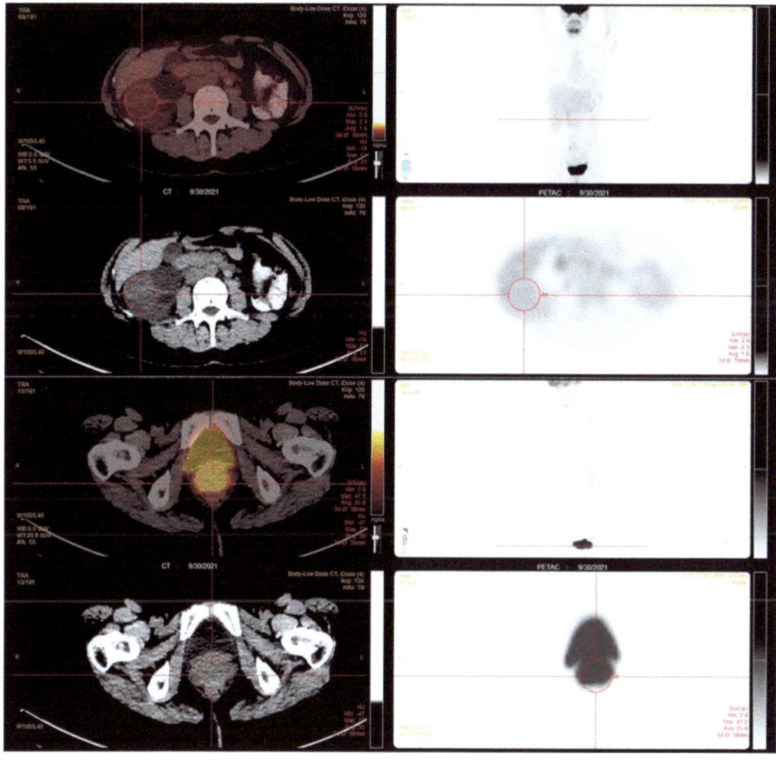

C. Y. O. Wong, D. Wu, *Phenotypic Oncology PET*,
https://doi.org/10.1007/978-3-031-09737-9_49

49.1   Case 49: Interpretation and Teaching

A1:   F-18 FDG.

A2:   Low FDG uptake is consistent with metabolic phenotype of RCC, while the high FDG uptake is consistent with metabolic phenotype of cervical cancer.

Teaching Point It's well known that renal clear cell carcinoma (RCC) has minimal to mild FDG activity, due to mucinous feature. In contrast, cervix cancer can show markedly increased metabolic activity, probably with contribution of inflammatory/reactive changes. Although many innovative radiotracers have been tested in RCC, robust differentiation of primary disease from normal parenchyma remains elusive for almost all of them. Since the evaluations of metastatic setting and response to therapy for this cancer are by far most important, FDG remains favorable PET tracer for clinical applications.

Reference

Lindenberg L, Mena E, Choyke PL, Bouchelouche K. PET imaging in renal cancer. Curr Opin Oncol. 2019;31(3):216–21.

Chapter 50
Case 50: Gallbladder Adenocarcinoma with Chemoresistance

A: Patient is a 73-year-old female undergoing initial staging PET-CT of biopsy-proven moderate to poorly differentiated gallbladder adenocarcinoma. (1) What is the tracer? (2) Did the gallbladder cancer invade liver parenchyma? (3) Is there any evidence for extrahepatic metastasis in the right abdomen?

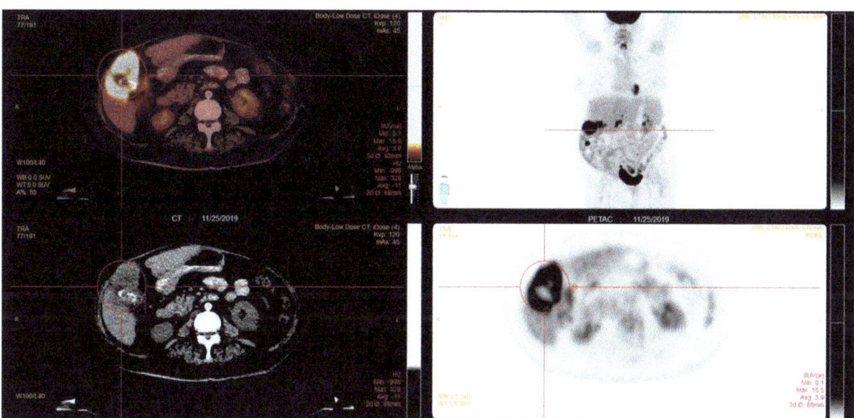

© The Author(s), under exclusive license to Springer Nature Switzerland AG 2022
C. Y. O. Wong, D. Wu, *Phenotypic Oncology PET*,
https://doi.org/10.1007/978-3-031-09737-9_50

B: Restaging PET-CT studies after 4 months (the upper panel) and 9 months (the lower panel) of chemotherapy. (1) How was the response initially and finally? (2) Was the cervix lesion primary or metastasis?

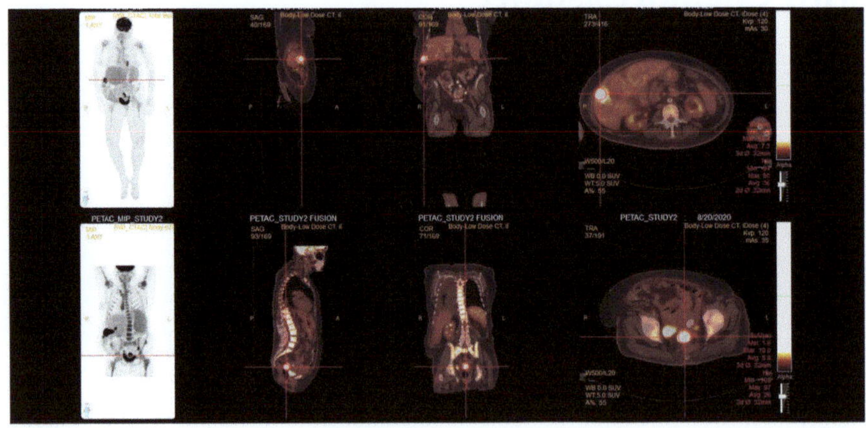

50.1 Case 50: Interpretation and Teaching

A1:   F-18 FDG.

A2:   It may invade into liver parenchyma which needs MRI confirmation.

A3:   There is an FDG-avid soft tissue lesion (MIP) in the right mid abdomen, suspicious for metastasis or seeding.

B1:   Initially there was a partial response, but final findings are highly suggestive of disease progression.

B2:   Due to new abnormal PET-CT findings, it is likely metastatic. A biopsy of the cervix lesion was performed, which was positive for metastasis of gallbladder adenocarcinoma.

Teaching Point Radical resection is offered to patients with nonmetastatic, invasive, incidental gallbladder cancer. It appears that in patients with incidental gallbladder cancer without metastatic disease, PET-CT and dedicated contrast CT seem to have roles complementing each other. PET-CT was able to detect occult metastatic or residual local-regional disease in some of these patients and seems to be useful in the preoperative diagnostic algorithm of patients whose CT is normal or indicates locally advanced disease.

Reference

Shukla PJ, Barreto SG, Arya S, et al. Does PET–CT scan have a role prior to radical re-resection for incidental gallbladder cancer? HPB (Oxford). 2008;10(6):439–45.

Chapter 51
Case 51: Wax-and-Wane Metabolic Activities of Low-Grade Lymphoma

A: Baseline and follow-up PET scans of biopsy proved mesenteric follicular lymphoma, grade 1, and CD20 and BCL positive. (1) What is the tracer? (2) Is there any evidence of FDG-avid lymphoma?

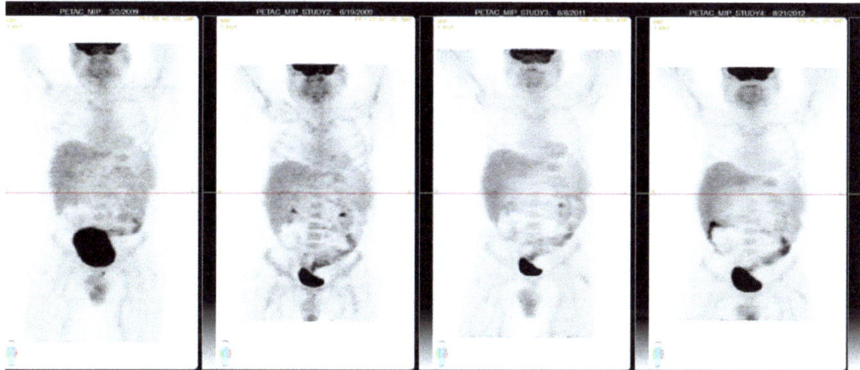

C. Y. O. Wong, D. Wu, *Phenotypic Oncology PET*,
https://doi.org/10.1007/978-3-031-09737-9_51

B. Continued follow-up PET. : (1) What is the new finding? (2) What's the appropriate recommendation?

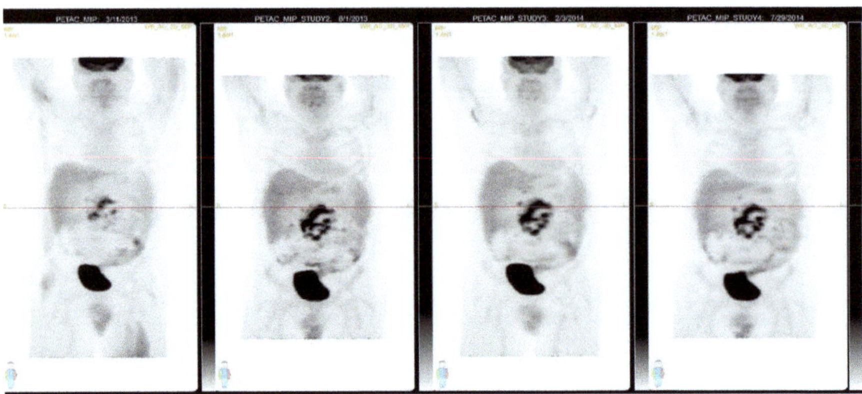

C. Further follow-up PET without therapy. : (1) What is the PET diagnosis? (2) What is the likely lymphoma phenotype?

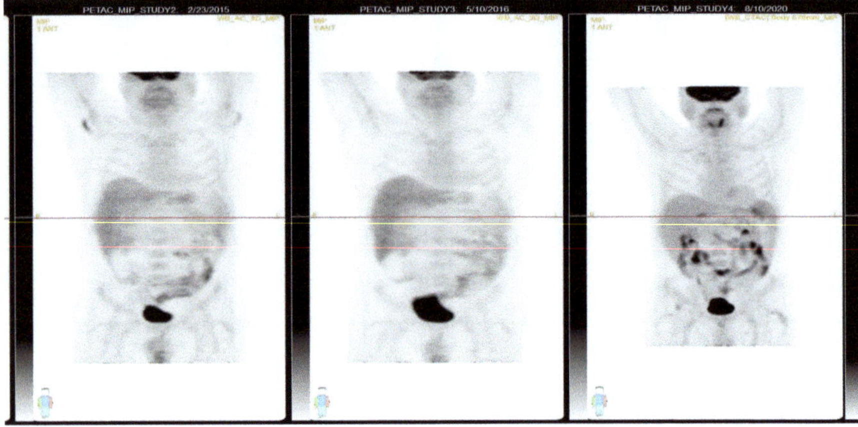

51.1   Case 51: Interpretation and Teaching

A1   F-18 FDG.

A2   No. There is no PET evidence of FDG-avid disease, but there is non-avid lymphoma.

Teaching Point 1 The concurrent CT showed mesenteric and retroperitoneal adenopathy and splenomegaly. The FDG PET negativity is consistent with the grade 1 follicular lymphoma phenotype.

B1   Conglomerate mesenteric and retroperitoneal adenopathy with steady increased FDG activities, max SUV 10.2 (prior max SUV 0.5–1.2), suggestive of disease progression.

B2   Possible malignant transformation prompts to recommend biopsy of the metabolically representative lesions shall be recommended. The pathology showed follicular lymphoma, grades 1–2.

Teaching Point 2 Maximal SUV greater than 15 or 3 times the baseline raises concern for transformation which may be missed on FNA or core biopsy. Therapy depends on symptoms.

C1   FDG activities wane on follow-up PET but there may still have non-avid low-grade lymphomas.

C2   Low-grade follicular lymphoma.

Teaching Point 3 It's notorious that low-grade follicular lymphoma can manifest spontaneous progression and remission, showing wax-and-wane metabolic activity on FDG PET. If search for excisional biopsy fails to reveal diffuse large B cell lymphoma (DLBCL), follow-up PET may provide information on possible malignant transformation.

Reference

Tang BT, Malysz J, Douglas-Nikitin V, et al. Correlating metabolic activity with cellular proliferation in follicular lymphomas. Mol Imaging Biol. 2009;11(5):296–302.

Chapter 52
Case 52: Reactive Adenopathy in Treated Classic Hodgkin's Lymphoma

A: Baseline PET (left panel) shows findings consistent with pathological diagnosis of classic Hodgkin's lymphoma confined to the right inguinal area and adjacent external iliac region with mild to moderate FDG activities, maximal SUV 5.2. Interim (middle panel, 2 months later) and post-chemotherapy (right panel, 6 months later) studies negative findings: (1) What is the tracer? (2) How was the response to chemotherapy?

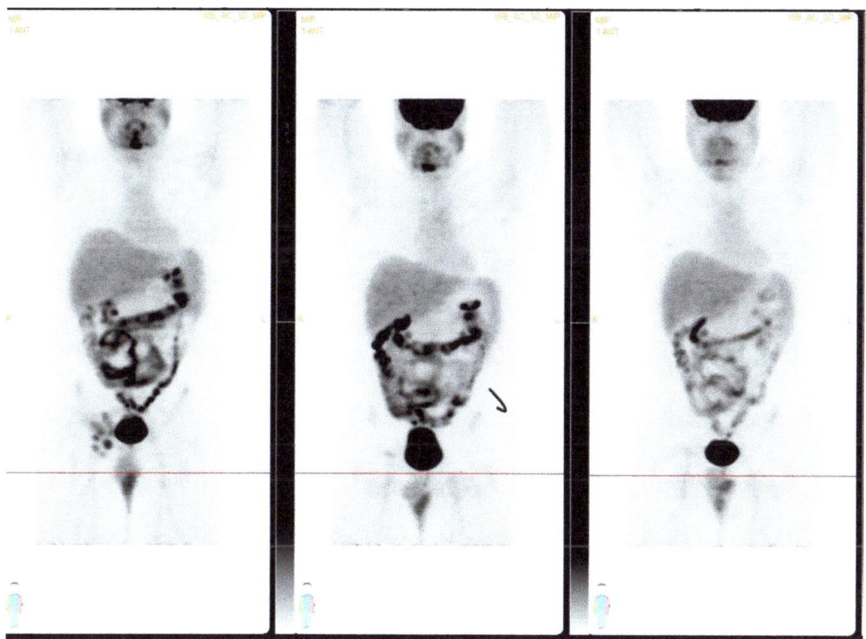

C. Y. O. Wong, D. Wu, *Phenotypic Oncology PET*,
https://doi.org/10.1007/978-3-031-09737-9_52

B. Further follow-up PET-CTs continue to show no discrete appreciable tracer activity in the right groin or pelvis. However, there is mild to moderate FDG activity corresponding to prominent lymph nodes in bilateral axilla, left greater than right side. (1) Is the FDG-avid left axillary node lymphoma? If not, why? (2) What's an appropriate recommendation?

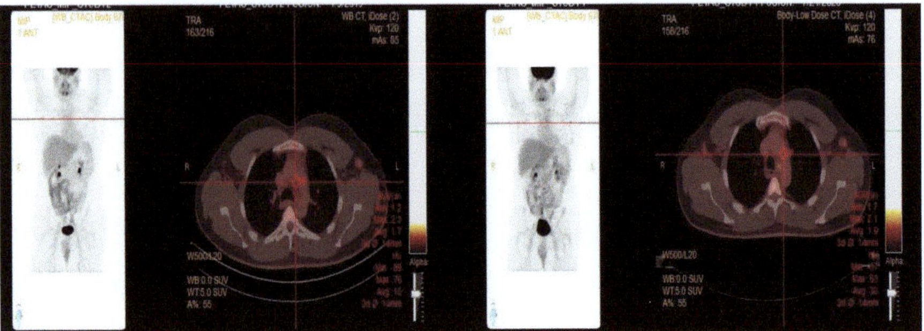

52.1 Case 52: Interpretation and Teaching

A1: F-18 FDG.

A2: The response to chemotherapy is excellent on the interim scan, with stable response on 6-month scan. Deauville 1–2.

B1: No. It is likely reactive.

Teaching Point 1 Classic Hodgkin's disease does not skip lesions. The baseline PET indicated stage II disease below the diaphragm. Recurrence after systemic therapy without local radiation usually occurs in the same site.

B2: Negative for recurrence; continual follow-up as indicated.

Teaching Point 2 Baseline PET is important in the involved field radiation. Recurrence occurs usually just outside the radiation field.

Reference

Figura N, Flampouri S, Mendenhall NP, et al. Importance of baseline PET/CT imaging on radiation field design and relapse rates in patients with Hodgkin lymphoma. Adv Radiat Oncol. 2017;2(2):197–203.

Chapter 53
Case 53: Chemo-Refractory DLBCL

A: Baseline PET-CT (left panel) shows findings consistent with pathological diagnosis of diffuse large B-cell lymphoma (DLBCL) via a core biopsy of left peritoneal/pancreatic mass, with extensive involvement of the spleen, and innumerous lymph nodes below and above the diaphragm. After treated with two cycles of R-CHOP, the patient underwent PET-CT (right panel) which shows all lesions above and below the diaphragm except for a lesion within the spleen, with enhanced tracer activity, current max SUV 36.2, compared to the prior max SUV 19.3 in the same splenic region. (1) What is the tracer? (2) What's the stage of DLBCL? (3) How was the response to chemotherapy, and what's Lugano score on the interim PET-CT?

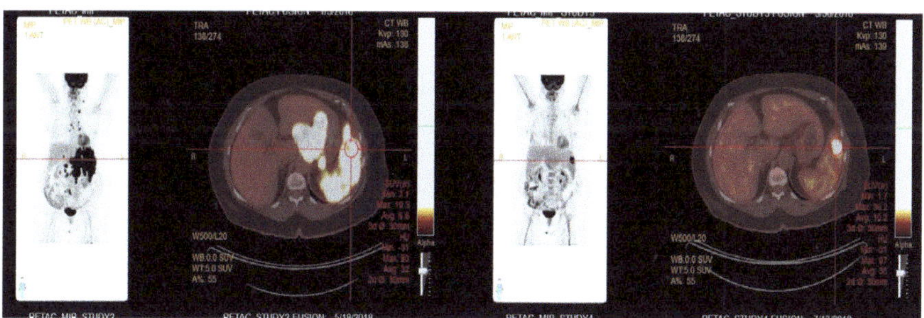

C. Y. O. Wong, D. Wu, *Phenotypic Oncology PET*,
https://doi.org/10.1007/978-3-031-09737-9_53

B. Biopsy of the splenic lesion revealed historically similar DLBCL, so the patient completed six cycles of R-CHOP as planned. Post-chemo PET-CT (right panel), however, showed a persistent splenic lesion, with mildly decreased tracer intensity, current max SUV 28.2, relative to prior max SUV 36.2. The left panel is a follow-up PET-CT after receiving three cycles of RICE as a salvage, which again showed a persistent splenic lesion, despite moderately decreased tracer intensity (current max SUV 6.8). (1) What are Lugano scores on the two follow-up PET-CT scans? (2) How is the prognosis of the patient?

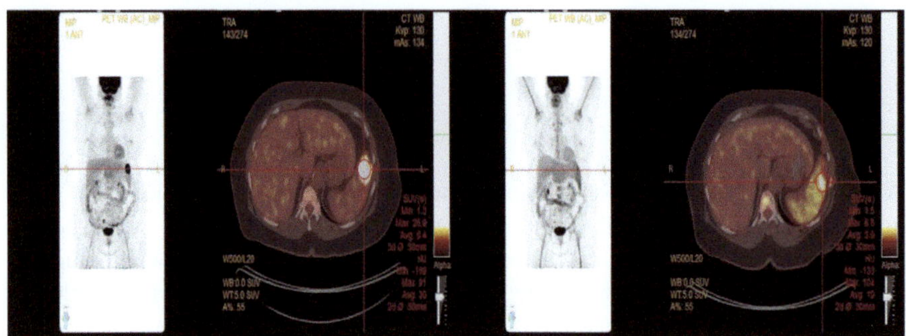

53.1 Case 53: Interpretation and Teaching

A1:   F-18 FDG.

A2:   The PET-CT findings are consistent with stage IIIs.

A3:   There is response to chemotherapy, but the overall response is not that favorable as it only partially responses after two cycles of R-CHOP. The persistent splenic lesion with even enhanced tracer activity is worrisome, as the Lugano score is at 5.

Teaching Point 1 Despite the overall unfavorable response to two-cycle R-CHOP, biopsy may be recommended for further workup of the persistent splenic lesion with even enhanced FDG activity, in hope of new historic and/or molecular/immunologic features to guide for more effective treatment.

B1:   The Lugano scores are 5 and 4, respectively.

The Lugano classification is a lymphoma staging system for non-Hodgkin's and Hodgkin's lymphoma. It outlines the classification for response to treatment based on PET-CT.

The Lugano classification recommends the Deauville 5-point scale for reporting response by FDG PET-CT:

1. No uptake or no residual uptake (when used interim).
2. Slight uptake but below blood pool (mediastinum).
3. Uptake above mediastinal but below or equal to uptake in the liver.
4. Uptake slightly to moderately higher than the liver.
5. Markedly increased uptake or any new lesion (on response evaluation).

Nonprogressive Disease
- Complete metabolic response (CMR).

  – Score of 1, 2, or 3 in nodal or extranodal sites with or without a residual mass.

- Partial metabolic response (PMR).

  – Score of 4 or 5 with reduced uptake compared with baseline and residual mass(es) of any size.

- Stable disease or no metabolic response.

  – Score of 4 or 5 with no obvious change in FDG uptake.

Progressive Disease
- Score of 4 or 5 in any lesion with an increase in intensity of FDG uptake from baseline (and/or new FDG-avid foci consistent with lymphoma).

Teaching Point 2 Chemo-refractory shall be considered, once patient fails a salvage treatment.

B2:   The prognosis of chemo-refractory lymphoma is usually very poor. Indeed, the patient passed away a few months after the last PET-CT study despite the salvage chemotherapy with RICE as aforementioned and reported autologous stem cell transplant (ASCT).

Reference

Vardhana SA, Sauter CS, Matasar MJ, Zelenetz AD, Galasso N, Woo KM, Zhang ZG, Moskowitz CH. Outcomes of primary refractory diffuse large B-cell lymphoma (DLBCL) treated with salvage chemotherapy and intention to transplant in the rituximab era. Br J Haematol. 2017;176(4):591–9.

Chapter 54
Case 54: Primary Cutaneous DLBCL, Leg Type (PC-DLBCL-LT)

A: Initial staging PET-CT was performed on this 88-year-old male who had a newly diagnosed diffuse large B-cell lymphoma (DLBCL) of left lower extremity. Curvilinear cutaneous and subcutaneous lesions are identified in the posterior and posterolateral of the left lower leg, abutting to but not definitely involving the calf muscle. Additionally, multiple spot cutaneous lesions are noted, lateral and inferior to the left knee joint, and bilateral distal left lower leg. The remainder of the whole-body PET-CT is essentially unremarkable, with special reference to the left popliteal and inguinal regions. (1) What is the tracer? (2) What's the PET diagnosis? (3) How is the prognosis?

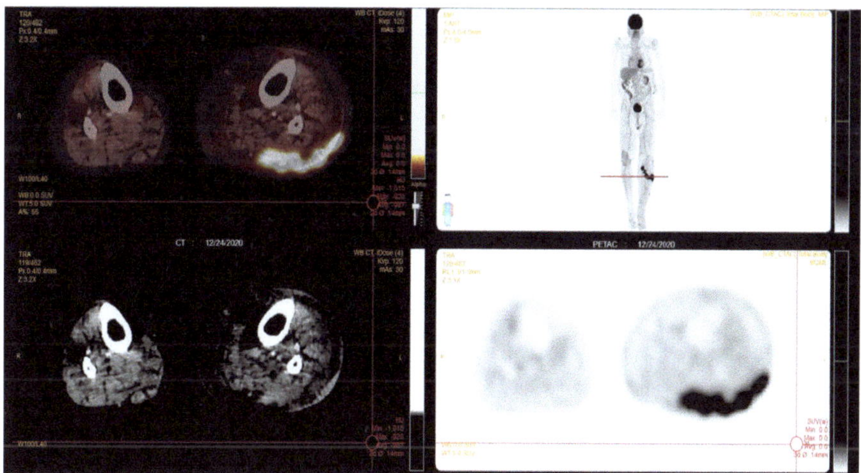

C. Y. O. Wong, D. Wu, *Phenotypic Oncology PET*,
https://doi.org/10.1007/978-3-031-09737-9_54

54.1   Case 54: Interpretation and Teaching

A1:   F-18 FDG.

A2:   Despite the lack of detailed pathology, the PET-CT findings are consistent with primary cutaneous diffuse large B-cell lymphoma, leg type (PCDLBCL-LT). The imaging features supporting the diagnosis include exclusive lymphomatous involvement of cutaneous or subcutaneous tissue in the left lower leg, but there is no underlying calf muscle invasion or bone, or nodal involvement particularly in the adjacent popliteal or inguinal areas.

Teaching Point   PCDLBCL-LT is a distinct entity of malignant lymphoma, and FDG PET-CT has the unique combined metabolic and anatomy features as afore-mentioned to help establish the diagnosis.

A3:   According to our clinical experience and limited literature, PC-DLBCL-LT often has a poor response to chemotherapy, probably due to decreased toler-ance from chemo-toxicity secondary to advanced age/comorbidity, limited blood perfusion to the far distal and peripheral tumor location, and finally the underlying pathological features as well as predisposed relapses. Advanced age, leg location, and multiple skin lesions are three most impor-tant predictive factors for death rate.

Reference

Patsatsi A, Kyriakou A, Karavasilis V, Panteliadou K, Sotiriadis D. Primary cutaneous diffuse large B-cell lymphoma, leg type, with multiple relapses: case presentation and brief review of literature. Hippokratia. 2013;17(2):174–6.

Chapter 55
Case 55: Primary Pulmonary MALT Lymphoma

A: Initial staging PET with newly diagnosed MALT (mucosa-associated lymphoid tissue) lymphoma shows multiple opacities in the right lung, all with moderate avidity, SUV 7.1 (RUL), 7.6 (RML), and 5.4 (RLL). The left lung is unremarkable. Note that there is mild tracer activity in the inferior left breast, corresponding to postsurgical changes (image not shown). There is no avid adenopathy in the mediastinum, hila, or axillae. The visualized portion of the head/neck and portion below the diaphragm are also unremarkable. (1) What is the tracer? (2) What is the PET diagnosis, and how is the prognosis?

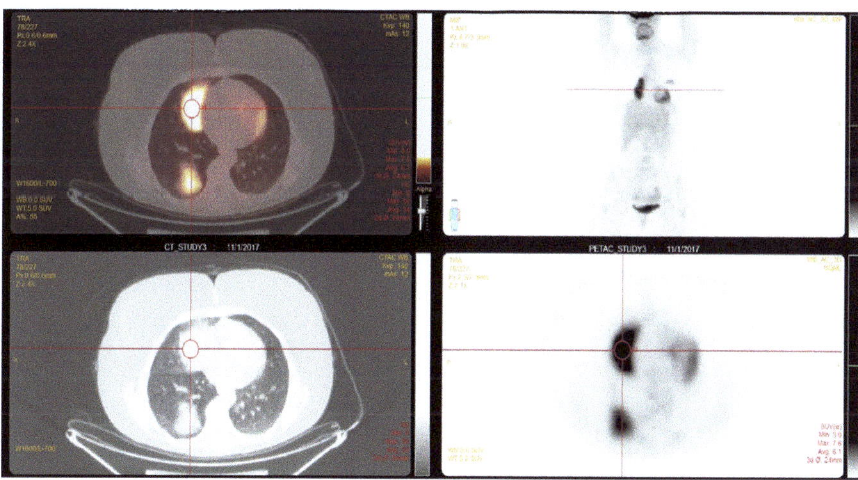

C. Y. O. Wong, D. Wu, *Phenotypic Oncology PET*,
https://doi.org/10.1007/978-3-031-09737-9_55

B. Interim (after two cycles of chemotherapy; the top panel) and completed chemotherapy (after six cycles, the bottom panel) PET-CT studies show complete resolution of the right lung lesions, without any appreciable tracer activity over background. Note that the previously mentioned focal mild tracer activity in the inferior left breast has also resolved, consistent with known postsurgical changes. (1) How was the response to chemotherapy, and what were the Lugano scores?

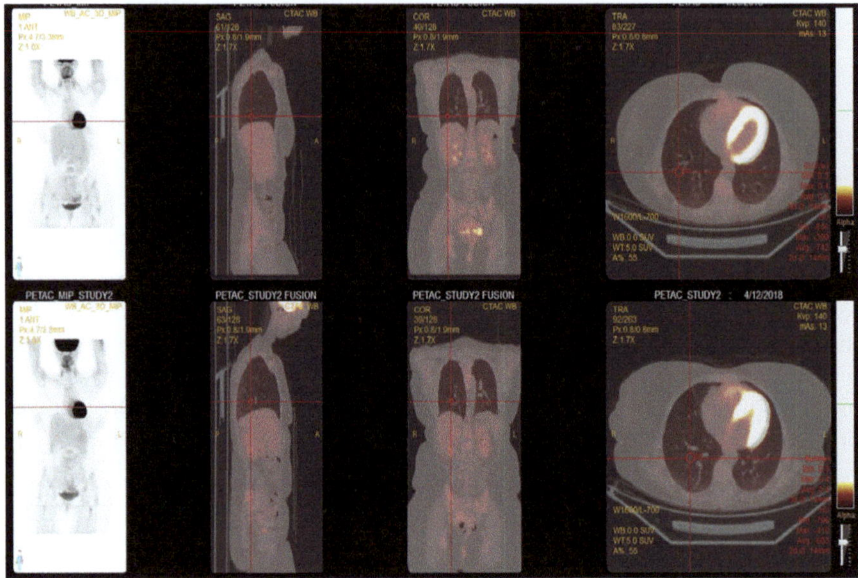

55.1   Case 55: Interpretation and Teaching

A1:   F-18 FDG.
A2:   The PET diagnosis is primary pulmonary MALT lymphoma, with an expected favorable prognosis.

Teaching Point   Primary pulmonary MALT is a less commonly diagnosed extranodal lymphoma but is the most frequent subset of primary pulmonary lymphoma. The median age at diagnosis is 50–60 years old. FDG PET-CT features support the diagnosis including one or multiple areas of infiltration/opacity, with mild to moderate FDG activity, exclusively in the lung parenchyma, without lymphonodular involvement in the hila, mediastinum, or elsewhere.

B1:   The response to chemotherapy was excellent, with Lugano scores of one on each of the two follow-up FDG PET-CT studies. A follow-up diagnostic CT performed 10 months after the last FDG PET-CT was also unremarkable and stable (data not shown), indicating a sustainable and favorable response to chemotherapy.

Reference

Bi L, Li J, Lu ZX. Pulmonary MALT lymphoma: a case report and review of the literature. Exp Ther Med. 2015;9:147–50.

Chapter 56
Case 56: Concurrent Low-Grade Follicular Lymphoma (LG FL) and DLBCL

A. Baseline PET was performed for initial staging of endoscopic biopsy-proved ileocecal and rectal mucosal low-grade follicular lymphoma, but SUV was 21.0. (1) What is the tracer? (2) Are PET-CT findings consistent with low-grade lymphoma? (3) What is the appropriate recommendation?

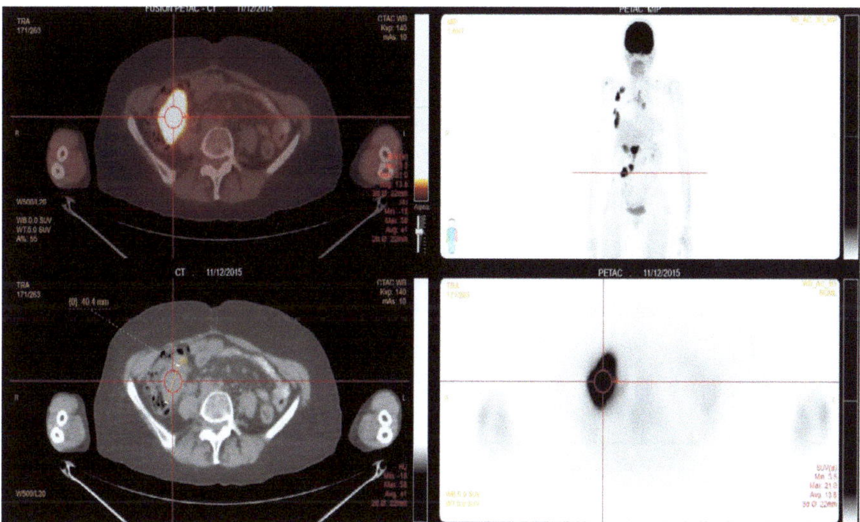

C. Y. O. Wong, D. Wu, *Phenotypic Oncology PET*,
https://doi.org/10.1007/978-3-031-09737-9_56

B. Post-chemotherapy follow-up PET (left two, interim and post-six-cycle R-CHOP, respectively; right two, prior and after two-cycle RICE, respectively). (1) How was the response to chemotherapies?

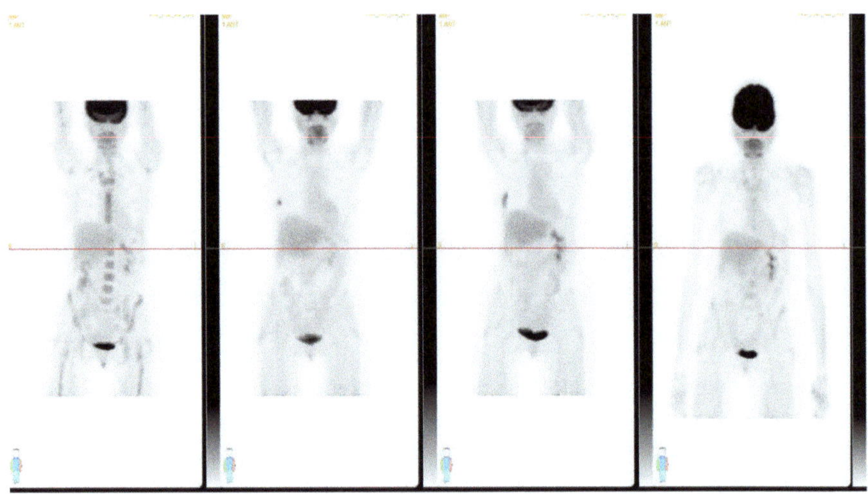

C. PET in two planes of coronal images showing chest wall recurrence (leftmost column in each coronal plane) and post-CART (chimeric antigen receptor T cells) (right three columns of each coronal plane). PET. (1) What was the response to immunotherapy? (2) What is the final PET-CT impression?

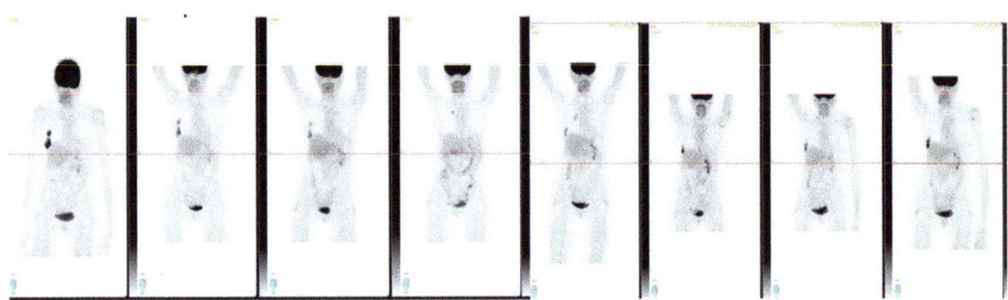

56.1 Case 56: Interpretation and Teaching

A1: F-18 FDG.

A2: No. Although some of the above-diaphragm nodes with mild FDG activity may represent low-grade lymphomas, conglomerate adenopathy in the right axilla and upper abdomen and the ileocecal mass (see crosshair) show intense activity, SUV 21.0, suggesting high-grade or transformed lymphoma.

A3: Biopsy (or better excision) of lesions with highest metabolic activity if possible is recommended.

Teaching Point Although biopsies often yield final and definite diagnosis, some of them may not necessarily represent the whole spectrum of the disease, due to limited tissue sampling, technical issues, and coexisting entities. Once discrepancy between PET imaging and pathology is noted, as demonstrated in this case, further workup including re-biopsy shall be recommended.

B1: Since excisional biopsy of right axillary node demonstrated diffuse large B-cell lymphoma (DLBCL) from a background of lowgrade follicular lymphoma, chemotherapy with R-CHOP was started that yielded a transient and partial response. The subsequent salvage chemotherapy with RICE resulted in a complete response.

C1: The patient underwent biopsy of the right chest wall lesion which was confirmed as recurrent DLBCL. The initial response to CART was steadily good over 1 year, but recurrent disease developed despite continued CART therapy during the further follow-up.

C2: The final PET impressions are concurrent low-grade follicular lymphoma and DLBCL, and the latter is chemoresistant and immuno-refractory.

Reference

Wang Y, Link BK, Witzig TE, et al. Impact of concurrent indolent lymphoma on the clinical outcome of newly diagnosed diffuse large B-cell lymphoma. Blood. 2019;134(16):1289–97.

Chapter 57
Case 57: Primary Bone Lymphoma (PBL)

A: Baseline PET-CT was performed for initial staging of newly diagnosed and biopsy-proven left scapular B-cell lymphoma. (1) What is the tracer? (2) What is the PET-CT impression?

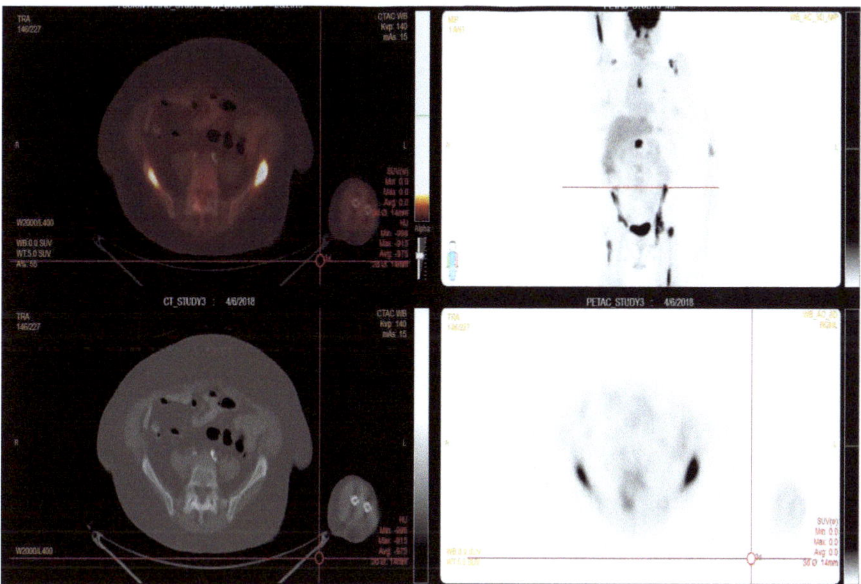

C. Y. O. Wong, D. Wu, *Phenotypic Oncology PET*, https://doi.org/10.1007/978-3-031-09737-9_57

B: Interim (after two cycles, the top panel) and post-chemotherapy (after six cycles, the bottom panel) follow-up PET-CT scans were performed with images as the following: (1) Why was the tracer activity T11 and L1 decreased? (2) What was the overall response to chemotherapy? (3) What is the prognosis?

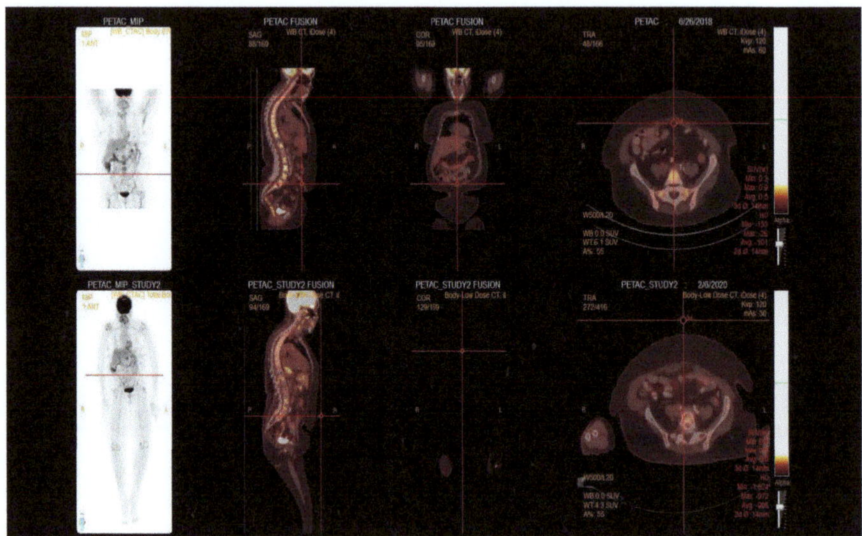

57.1   Case 57: Interpretation and Teaching

A1:   F-18 FDG.

A2:   The PET-CT impression is primary bone lymphoma (PBL), as multiple FDG-avid lesions, all with no definite CT correlate or with minimal sclerotic changes, are identified, exclusively involving multiple sites of the bone or bone marrow, including at least bilateral scapula (with left being biopsy proven), left humerus, the sternum, T11 and L1, bilateral iliac bones, the right sacrum, and bilateral proximal femurs.

Teaching Point 1   PBL is characterized by exclusive or predominant lymphomatous involvement of the bone or bone marrow. According to our clinical experience and limited literature, all PBLs are DLBCL, though pathology may or may not yield the final diagnosis due to a variety of reasons.

B1:   The decreased FDG activity at T11 and L1 is indicating treated lymphoma, while the adjacent vertebral bodies with increased FDG activity is most likely due to normal marrow with reactive changes to chemotherapy.

B2:   The response to chemotherapy was excellent, with Lugano score of 1–2.

B3:   The patient achieved a complete remission, with an excellent prognosis.

Teaching Point 2   PBL is a distinct entity, and the use of Lugano score for evaluation of treatment response needs caution about the potential of persistent residual activity after successful treatment especially for lesions near joints and a lack of comparison to contralateral and adjacent normal bone or bone marrow due to reactive changes to chemotherapy. Extended longitudinal PET-CT follow-up to establish interval stability is a good option, given the good long-term prognosis of PBL.

Reference

Beal K, Allen L, Yahalom J. Primary bone lymphoma: treatment results and prognostic factors with long-term follow-up of 82 patients. Cancer. 2006;106(12):2652–6.

Chapter 58
Case 58: Lymphomatoid Granulomatosis (LYG) Variant of DLBCL

A: Baseline PET-CT (left panel) was performed for initial staging of biopsy-proven left upper and lower lung DLBCL, Epstein-Barr virus (EBV) positive. (1) What is the tracer? (2) What is the PET-CT impression? (3) Any incidental CT findings of significance?

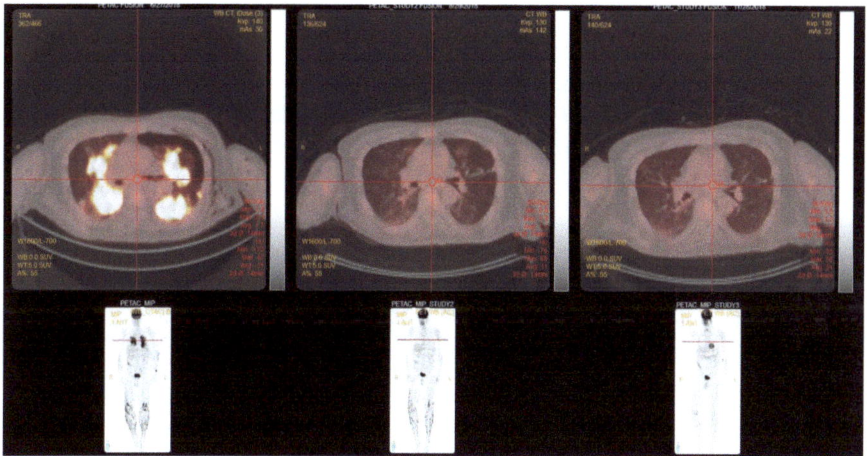

B: Interim (after two cycles of R-CHOP, the middle panel) and post-chemotherapy (after 6 cycles of R-CHOP, the right panel) follow-up PET-CT scans were performed with images as displayed above. (1) How was the initial response based on the interim PET-CT, and what was the Lugano score? (2) What was an appropriate recommendation? (3) What were the final response and Lugano score?

C. Y. O. Wong, D. Wu, *Phenotypic Oncology PET*, https://doi.org/10.1007/978-3-031-09737-9_58

58.1   Case 58: Interpretation and Teaching

A1:   F-18 FDG.

A2:   Lymphomatoid granulomatosis (LYG) variant of DLBCL is supported by biopsy-proven DLBCL with diffuse bilateral lung involvement SUV 23.0, and innumerous skin/cutaneous nodules involving bilateral upper and lower extremities, LE > UE, with mild to moderate metabolic activity.

A3:   Yes, the concurrent CT showed a moderate-sized left pneumothorax and left chest wall subcutaneous emphysema, which is apparently a sequela of recent left lung biopsies. The referring physician shall be contacted immediately with the incident CT findings of clinical significance for appropriate management or treatment if needed.

Teaching Point 1 Lymphomatoid granulomatosis (LYG) variant of DLBCL is a rare EBV-associated angio-centric and angio-destructive lymphoproliferative disease, often diffusely involving the lung and the cutaneous tissues of the extremities. This PET-CT study shows all the imaging features, in conjunction with the pathology findings, to support the diagnosis.

B1:   The initial response in the lungs was excellent but was partial in the upper and lower extremities, with a Lugano score 4.

B2:   Therefore, biopsy of the skin/cutaneous lesions shall be recommended. Indeed, a punch biopsy of right forearm skin lesion confirmed cutaneous lymphomatoid granulomatosis (LYG).

B3:   Continued R-CHOP treatment resulted in a complete response and final Lugano score of 1–2.

Reference

Sukswai N, Lyapichev K, Khoury JD, Medeiros LJ. Lymphoma 2020 update: diffuse large B-cell lymphoma variants. Pathology. 2020;52(1):53–67.

Chapter 59
Case 59: Secondary CNS Lymphoma

A: Baseline PET-CT (the far-left panel) was performed for initial staging of biopsy-proven DLBCL. Follow-up PET scans (second to fourth from left to right) were listed for interim, 1 and 6 months after completion of chemotherapy, respectively. (1) What is the tracer? (2) How was the initial response to chemotherapy? (3) Did the 6-month post-therapy study (far-right panel) show new findings in the left chest?

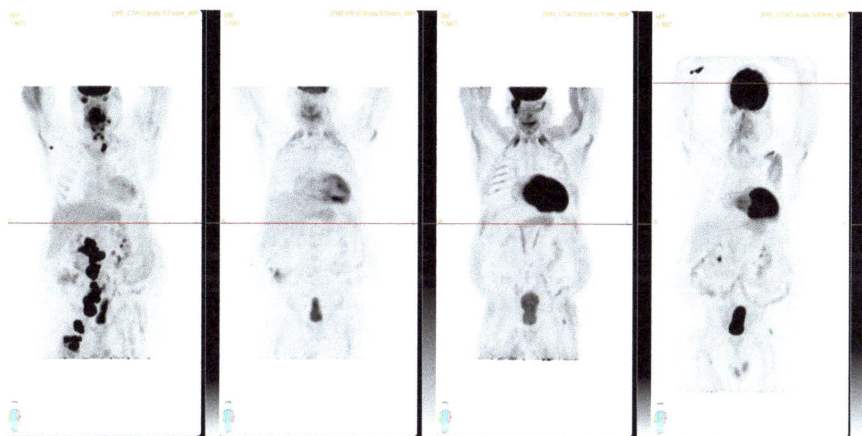

© The Author(s), under exclusive license to Springer Nature Switzerland AG 2022

C. Y. O. Wong, D. Wu, *Phenotypic Oncology PET*, https://doi.org/10.1007/978-3-031-09737-9_59

B: Due to newly developed aphasia and headache, whole brain was included as part of the most recent PET-CT study (far-right panel), and dedicated brain PET-CT images are displayed as the following: (1) What's PET-CT impression of the left-brain lesion? (2) What's an appropriate recommendation?

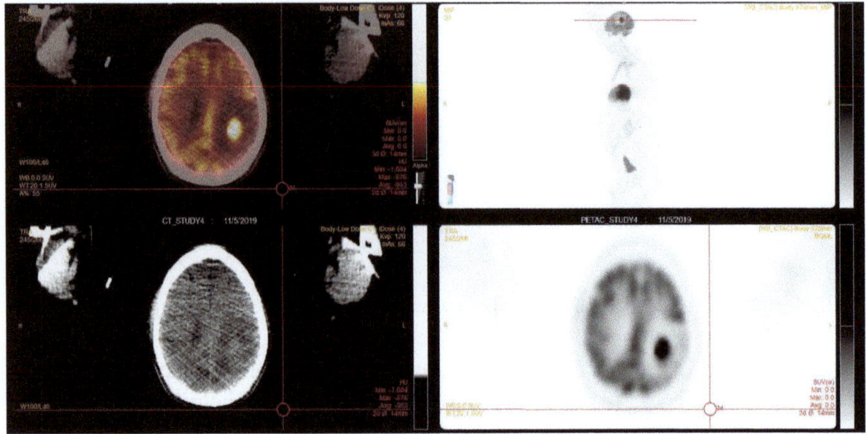

59.1   Case 59: Interpretation and Teaching

A1:   F-18 FDG.

A2:   The initial response to chemotherapy was favorable, as evidenced by resolved FDG-avid adenopathy below and above the diaphragm, although nonspecific findings were indicating labored respiration and right facial muscle uptake.

A3:   However, the 6-month post-therapy study shows new FDG-avid adenopathy in the left supraclavicular and subpectoral regions, suspicious for recurrent lymphoma.

B1:   Additionally, the brain/head scan revealed a moderate-sized focal increased FDG activity corresponding to a soft tissue mass in the left posterior frontal lobe, surrounded by decreased FDG activity, highly suspicious for a tumor with mass effects and vasogenic edema.

B2:   Although the PET-CT findings are highly abnormal, correlation with MRI brain is recommended with subsequent biopsy of the left posterior frontal mass that revealed DLBCL.

Teaching Point Secondary CNS lymphoma is a significant development in non-Hodgkin's lymphoma patients, due to the needs of intrathecal chemotherapy and a poor prognosis. Whole brain/head scan shall be included in addition to routine in PET-CT oncology imaging protocol, once patients report neurological symptoms. MRI brain and/or biopsy is recommended for abnormal PET-CT findings in brain parenchyma for further anatomic imaging characterization and/or definite tissue diagnosis.

Reference

Jahnke K, Thiel E, Martus P, et al. Retrospective study of prognosis factors in non-Hodgkin lymphoma secondarily involving the central nervous system. Ann Hematol. 2006;85:45–50.

Chapter 60
Case 60: Discordant PET in Low-Grade B-Cell Lymphoma

A: Baseline PET-CT was performed for initial staging of biopsy-proven left neck low-grade B-cell lymphoma. (1) What is the tracer? (2) Were PET-CT findings consistent with pathological diagnosis of low-grade lymphoma? (3) What's an appropriate recommendation?

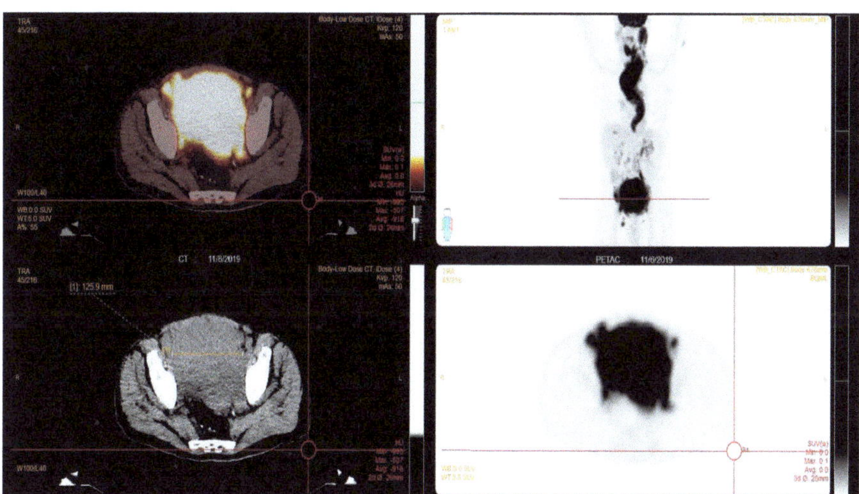

C. Y. O. Wong, D. Wu, *Phenotypic Oncology PET*,
https://doi.org/10.1007/978-3-031-09737-9_60

B: Interim (after two cycles of R-CHOP, the middle panel) and post-chemotherapy (after six cycles of R-CHOP, the right panel) follow-up PET-CT scans were performed with images as the following: (1) How was the response to chemotherapy, and what was the Lugano score?

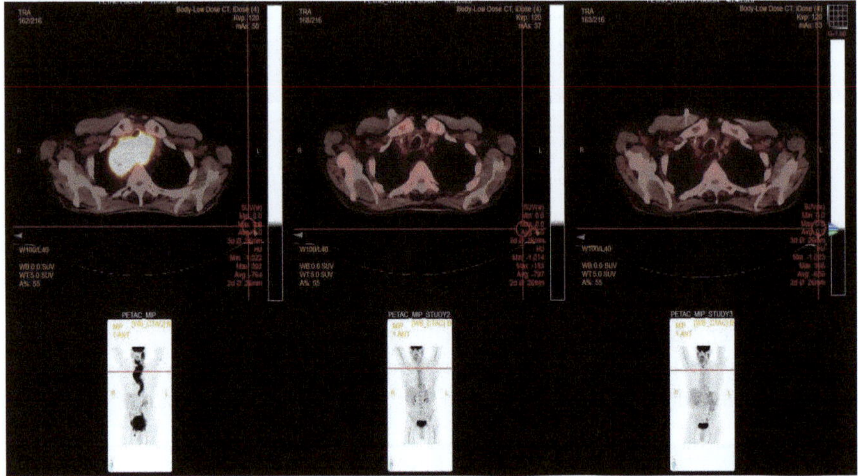

60.1 Case 60: Interpretation and Teaching

A1:   F-18 FDG.

A2:   No. In addition to the known left neck mass with abnormal FDG activity, there is diffuse involvement of the entire esophagus with mass formation in the upper and middle portions. Also, there is an approximately 13 cm urinary bladder mass with abnormal FDG activity, and the massive extranodal involvement of the esophagus and bladder is indicating malignant high-grade rather than low-grade lymphoma.

A3:   Due to the discrepancy between PET-CT and pathology, biopsy of the upper esophagus or the urinary bladder mass for definite diagnosis is highly recommended.

Teaching Point In addition to the massive involvement of the entire esophagus, the 13 cm FDG-avid urinary bladder mass is considered as bulky disease, which is an indicator for consultation for potential consolidation radiation therapy as a part of the treatment protocol.

B1:   The patient did not undergo any biopsy despite the apparent discordant PET-CT findings. Instead, the patient received treatment for aggressive lymphoma for a total of six-cycle R-CHOP for presumed transformed lymphoma. The response to chemotherapy was favorable, with a Lugano score of 1–2.

Reference

Jerusalem G, Beguin Y, Najjar F, et al. Positron emission tomography (PET) with 18F-fluorodeoxyglucose (18F-FDG) for the staging of low-grade non-Hodgkin's lymphoma (NHL). Ann Oncol. 2001;12(6):825–30.

Chapter 61
Case 61: Transplant-Related B-Cell Lymphoma

A: Baseline PET-CT (the far-left panel) was performed for initial staging of cytology-proven B-cell lymphoma, via positive FNA of subcarinal and right supraclavicular lymph nodes. (1) What is the tracer? (2) The patient was status post-liver transplant due to alcohol abuse and HCV. Single-agent therapy with Rituxan was administered, and three follow-up PET-CT scans were performed during the ensuing half a year as listed below. How was the response to therapy in terms of lesions above and below the diaphragm? (3) What is the Lugano score?

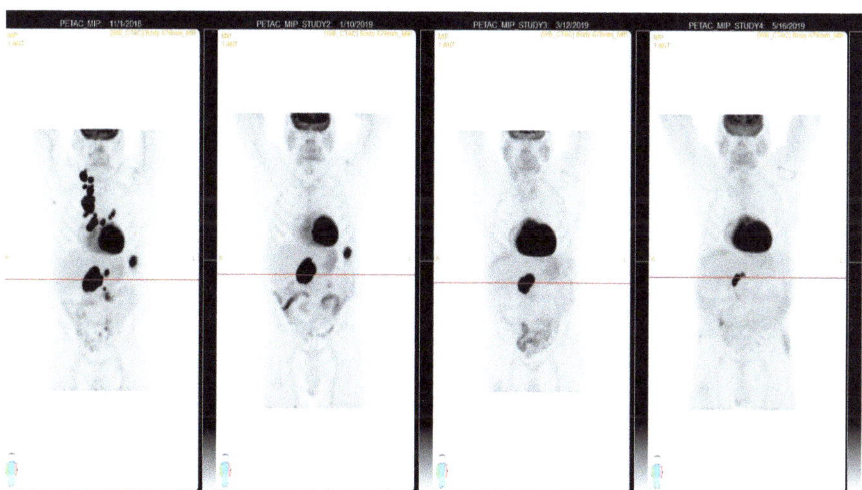

199

C. Y. O. Wong, D. Wu, *Phenotypic Oncology PET*,
https://doi.org/10.1007/978-3-031-09737-9_61

B: Due to the failed single-agent therapy, patient received four cycles of mini-R-CHOP, and subsequent follow-up PET-CTs were performed with images listed as the following: (1) What causes the bone marrow uptake on the first PET-CT following mini-R-CHOP? (2) What is the likely cause of the increased FDG activities in the left shoulder region? (3) What's final Lugano score?

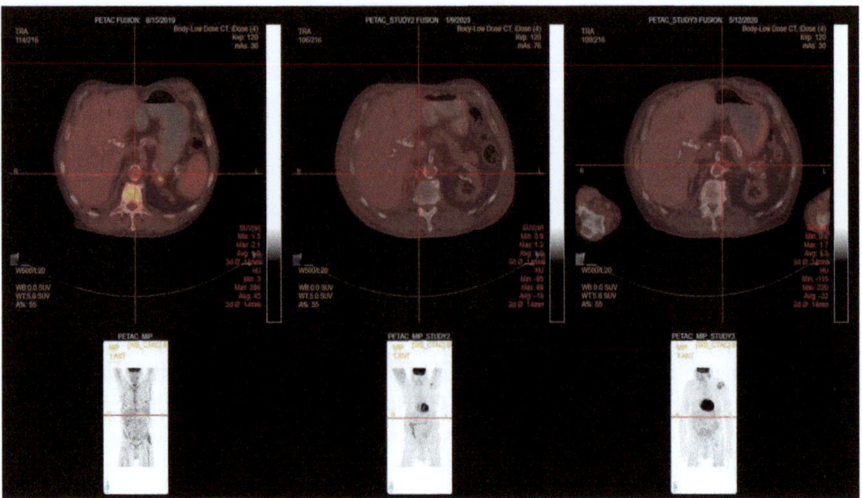

61.1   Case 61: Interpretation and Teaching

A1:   F-18 FDG.

A2:   The single-agent therapy with Rituxan resulted in complete remission of lymphomas above the diaphragm, but it had lesser effect on multiple lesions below diaphragm including one splenic lesion. The therapeutical efficacy looks like in the following order: lesions above diaphragm > splenic lesion > portocaval nodes.

A3:   The Lugano score is 5 due to persistent portocaval nodes with markedly increased FDG activity compared to the liver.

Teaching Point 1   It's well known that abdominal lymphomas are often less sensitive to chemotherapy when compared to lymphomas above the diaphragm such as mediastinal lymphomas.

B1:   The diffuse and symmetric FDG activity in bone marrow is most likely due to reactive changes to chemo agents, which was subsided on the further follow-up studies.

B2:   The steady increased FDG activity in the left shoulder region is likely due to arthritic changes. Clinical correlation is recommended if indicated.

B3:   The final Lugano score is 1.

Teaching Point 2   Rituximab (Rituxan) has been increasingly used as a highly effective therapeutic agent for both indolent and aggressive CD-20 positive B-cell lymphoma.

Reference

Dotan E, Aggarwal C, Smith MR. Impact of rituximab (Rituxan) on the treatment of B-cell non-Hodgkin's lymphoma. P T. 2010;35(3):148–57.

Chapter 62
Case 62: Bone Lesions in Primary Breast Lymphoma

A: Baseline PET-CT staging of biopsy-proven left breast diffuse large B-cell lymphoma (DLBCL) favored germinal center subtype. Bone marrow biopsy prior to PET-CT was negative. (1) What is the tracer? (2) What were the bone lesions? Why? (3) Is a repeated marrow biopsy necessary?

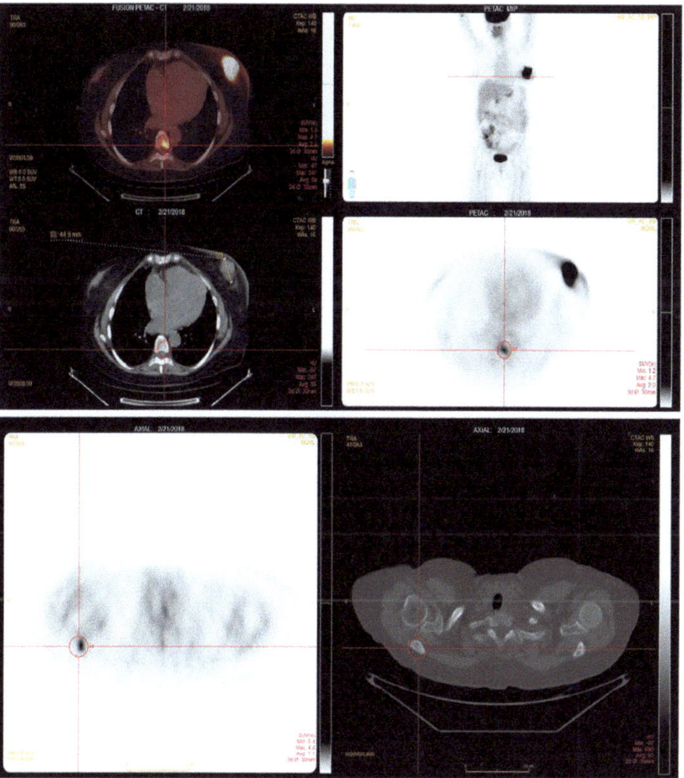

C. Y. O. Wong, D. Wu, *Phenotypic Oncology PET*,
https://doi.org/10.1007/978-3-031-09737-9_62

B: After four cycles, R-CHOP was stopped due to toxicity, and follow-up PET-CTs were performed 4 and 12 months (left two panels) since the baseline study, respectively. PET-CT (the third panel, 18 months) showed extensive liver lesions with biopsy positive for recurrent DLBCL. After three cycles of RICE, PET-CT was performed (far-right panel). (1) How was the initial response to chemotherapy? (2) Why was the relapse a surprise?

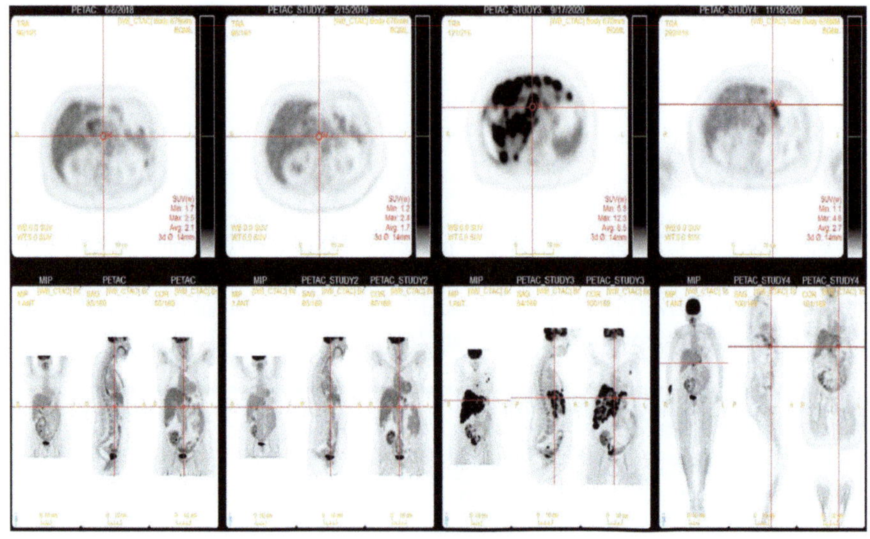

62.1   Case 62: Interpretation and Teaching

A1:   F-18 FDG.
A2:   The FDG-avid bone lesions are assumed lymphoma despite negative bone marrow biopsy (BMBx). Imaging features supporting the diagnosis of lymphoma include multiple sites (left T7, right scapula, and bilateral humerus) and lytic changes at the right scapula in addition to focal FDG avidity.
A3:   A repeated BMBx is unnecessary; therefore, it is not recommended.

Teaching Point 1 With focal lesion(s) in FDG PET-CT or MRI, routine BMBx for staging of lymphoma is not recommended.

B1:   The initial response to chemotherapy was favorable, as evidenced by markedly decreased FDG activity at the left breast primary site, and resolution of all the bone or bone marrow lesions, with a Lugano score of 1–2.
B2:   However, recurrence occurred 1 year since the initial chemotherapy, which is not a surprise, given the history of high-grade breast lymphoma phenotype and bone involvement despite negative bone marrow biopsy.

Teaching Point 2 Primary breast lymphoma is a rare malignancy that accounts for only 1% of malignant breast neoplasms. As shown in this case, primary breast lymphoma is characterized by a breast mass, without even axillary lymph nodal involvement, though bone or bone marrow involvement is obvious.

Reference

Gupta V, Bhutani N, Singh S, et al. Primary non-Hodgkin's lymphoma of breast—a rare cause of breast lump. Human Pathology: Case Reports. 2017;7:47–50.

Chapter 63
Case 63: FDG-Avid Recurrent GIST with Necrosis

A: Restaging PET-CT was performed for evaluation of known GIST, followed by separate IV contrasted CT. (1) What is the tracer? (2) What is likely grade of the GIST? (3) What is the usual targeted treatment and how-to follow-up?

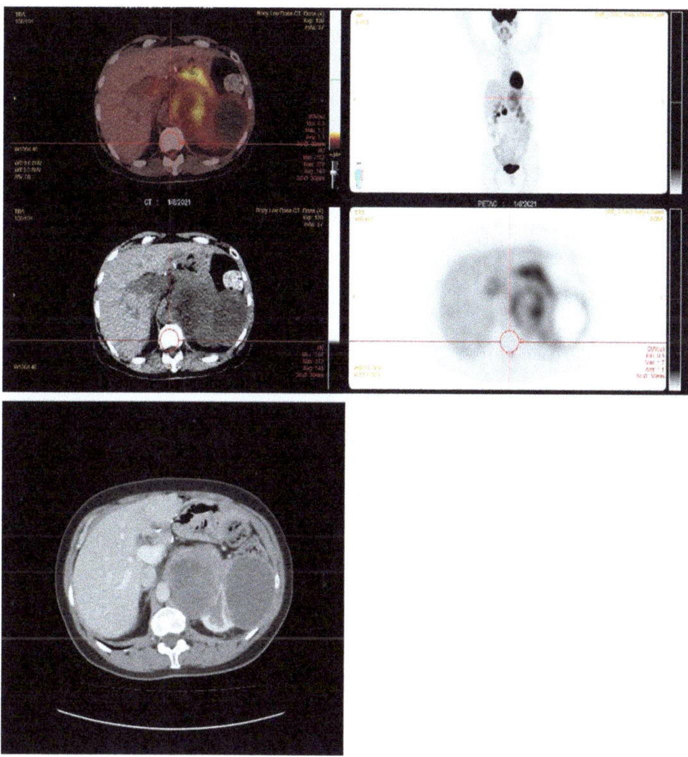

C. Y. O. Wong, D. Wu, *Phenotypic Oncology PET*,
https://doi.org/10.1007/978-3-031-09737-9_63

63.1 Case 63: Interpretation and Teaching

A1:   F-18 FDG.

A2:   Despite the necrotic component, there is active metabolism around the solid comportment and around the rim to suggest high-grade type.

A3:   Thymidine kinase inhibitor such as Gleevec is usually employed as the preferred first treatment, and PET-CT should be scheduled close to the end of each treatment as the GIST may rebound.

Teaching Point The therapy with tyrosine kinase inhibitors such as Gleevec and other targeted therapies in GIST may lead only to a minor tumor volume reduction even in cases of response. Therefore, the use of CT has limitations. FDG PET-CT is helpful for the assessment of early therapy response at the appropriate time intervals for therapy monitoring. Clinical response to treatment with small molecular inhibitor is predicted by KIT mutation status.

Reference

Dimitrakopoulou-Strauss A, Ronellenfitsch U, Cheng C, et al. Imaging therapy response of gastrointestinal stromal tumors (GIST) with FDG PET, CT and MRI: a systematic review. Clin Transl Imaging. 2017;5:183–97.

Chapter 64
Case 64: Metabolic Phenotypes in Peritoneal Mesothelioma

A: Staging PET-CT with newly diagnosed peritoneal mesothelioma. (1) What is the tracer? (2) What is the PET diagnosis, and how is the prognosis?

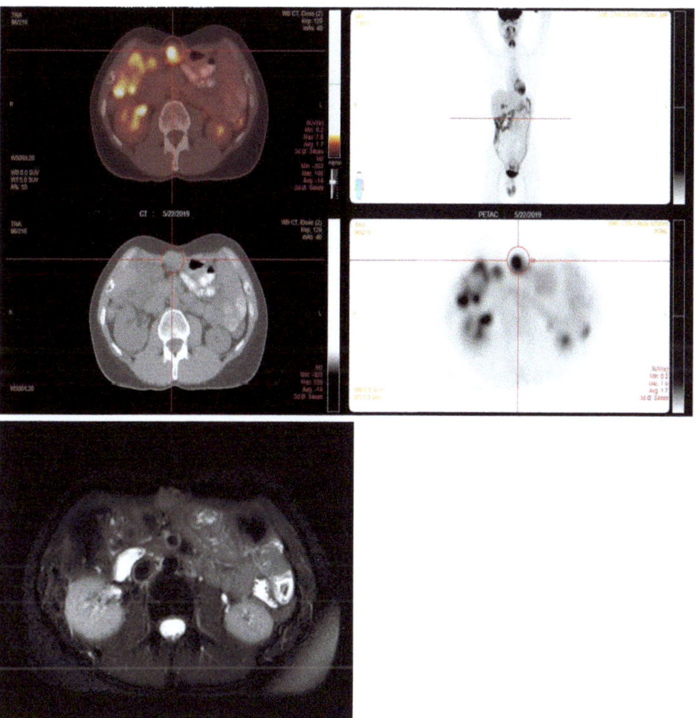

C. Y. O. Wong, D. Wu, *Phenotypic Oncology PET*,
https://doi.org/10.1007/978-3-031-09737-9_64

64.1 Case 64: Interpretation and Teaching

A1:   F-18 FDG.

A2:   The PET diagnosis is peritoneal carcinomatosis, with an expected poor prognosis.

Teaching Point Multicystic peritoneal mesothelioma histology was significantly associated with lower metabolic phenotype (SUV) compared to the epithelioid peritoneal mesothelioma.

Recurrences are common in the epithelioid peritoneal mesothelioma, whereas few recurrences are observed among multicystic peritoneal mesothelioma patients. The SUV of the lesions and patients' age are significantly associated with progression-free survival (PFS) in patients with epithelioid peritoneal mesothelioma.

Reference

Dubreuil J, Giammarile F, Rousset P, et al. The role of 18F-FDG-PET/ce CT in peritoneal mesothelioma. Nucl Med Commun. 2017;38(4):312–8.

Chapter 65
Case 65: Cutaneous Kaposi Sarcoma

A: Truncated FDG PET-CT was performed for Kaposi sarcoma

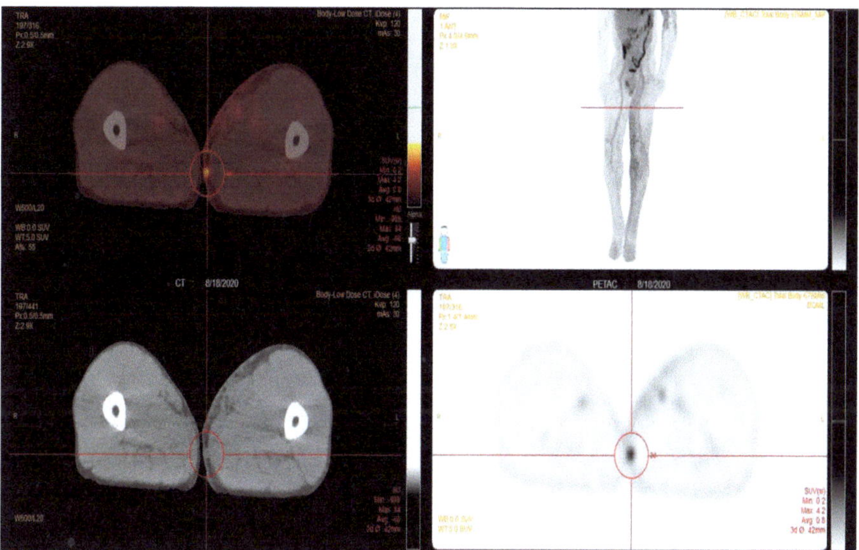

C. Y. O. Wong, D. Wu, *Phenotypic Oncology PET*,
https://doi.org/10.1007/978-3-031-09737-9_65

B:. Physical examination with a color photo showing patient's cutaneous Kaposi sarcomas of left upper extremity. (1) What is the tracer? (2) Were PET-CT findings consistent with cutaneous Kaposi sarcoma?

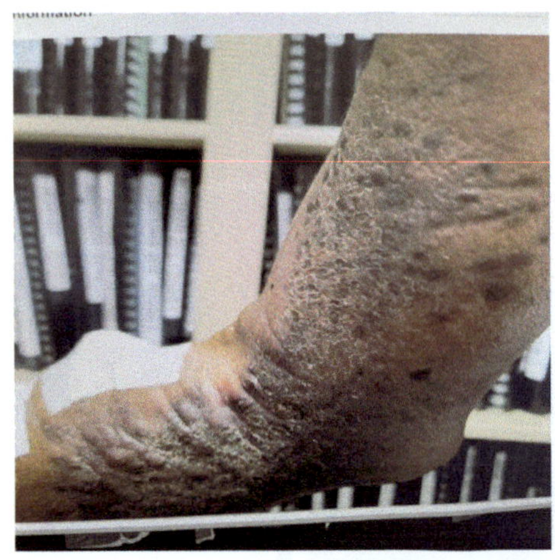

65.1   Case 65: Interpretation and Teaching

B1:   F-18 FDG.
B2:   FDG PET CT findings are consistent with cutaneous Kaposi sarcomas with mild to moderate metabolic activities.

Teaching Point   The skin and subcutaneous tissues are common sites of inflammatory lesions such as acne, sebaceous cysts, warts, and pilonidal cyst which may be FDG avid and/or abnormalities on the CT. However, the skin may be also the site of primary malignancies such as melanoma, squamous cell carcinoma, Kaposi sarcoma, lymphoma, or metastases. It is usually not possible to distinguish these benign and malignant lesions on whole-body FDG PET-CT. Fortunately, the skin allows for direct inspection of abnormalities. Thus, often the best method for further evaluation of abnormality seen on FDG PET-CT is the suggestion to perform a physical examination to correlate with imaging findings. Usually the patient is no longer available to the radiologist when a skin or subcutaneous lesion is identified on PET-CT images. In clinics where the patient is available to the interpreting radiologist, this is one abnormality where the radiologist can perform their own physical examination. More often it is done by referring physician in view of FDG PET-CT.

Reference

Polizzotto MN, Millo C, Uldrick TS, et al. F18-fluorodeoxyglucose Positron Emission Tomography in Kaposi Sarcoma Herpesvirus–Associated Multicentric Castleman Disease: Correlation With Activity, Severity, Inflammatory and Virologic Parameters. J Infect Dis. 2015;212:1250–60.

Chapter 66
Case 66: FDG-Avid Active Myeloma

A: Staging PET-CT was performed for myeloma. (1) What is the tracer? (2) What is the PET-CT impression? (3) How does PET impact treatment?

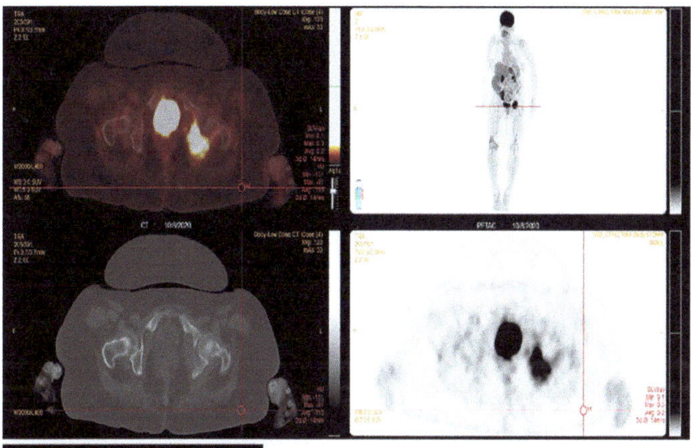

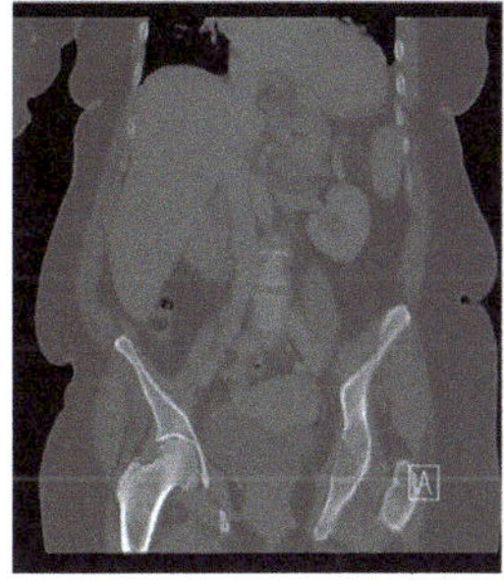

© The Author(s), under exclusive license to Springer Nature Switzerland AG 2022

C. Y. O. Wong, D. Wu, *Phenotypic Oncology PET*, https://doi.org/10.1007/978-3-031-09737-9_66

66.1 Case 66: Interpretation and Teaching

A1: F-18 FDG.
A2: The PET-CT impression is active myeloma or plasmacytoma.
A3: Active lesions warrant aggressive treatment.

Teaching Point ^{18}F-FDG PET-CT is indicated for both newly diagnosed and relapsed or refractory multiple myeloma because it assesses bone damage with relatively high sensitivity and specificity and detects extramedullary sites of proliferating clonal plasma cells while providing important prognostic information.

[8]F-FDG PET-CT is mandatory to confirm a suspected diagnosis of solitary plasmacytoma. The whole-body MRI is not always feasible to perform and to distinguish between smoldering and active multiple myeloma if whole-body X-ray (WBXR) is negative.

^{18}F-FDG PET-CT can distinguish between metabolically active and inactive disease which is the preferred functional imaging modality to monitor therapy on myeloma cell metabolism. Changes in FDG avidity can provide an earlier evaluation of response to therapy compared to MRI scans and can predict outcomes, particularly for those eligible to receive autologous stem cell transplantation.

^{18}F-FDG PET-CT can be coupled with sensitive bone marrow-based techniques to detect minimal residual disease (MRD) inside and outside the bone marrow, helping to identify and define those having imaging MRD negativity.

Reference

Cavo M, Terpo SE, Nanni C, et al. Role of [18] F-FDG PET/CT in the diagnosis and management of multiple myeloma and other plasma cell disorders: a consensus statement by the international myeloma working group. Lancet Oncol. 2017;18(4):e206–17.

Chapter 67
Case 67: Pancreatic Cancer with Abdominopelvic Carcinomatosis

A: The staging PET for known pancreatic cancer. (1) What is the tracer? (2) What is the PET-CT impression? (3) Any evidence for metastasis above the diagram?

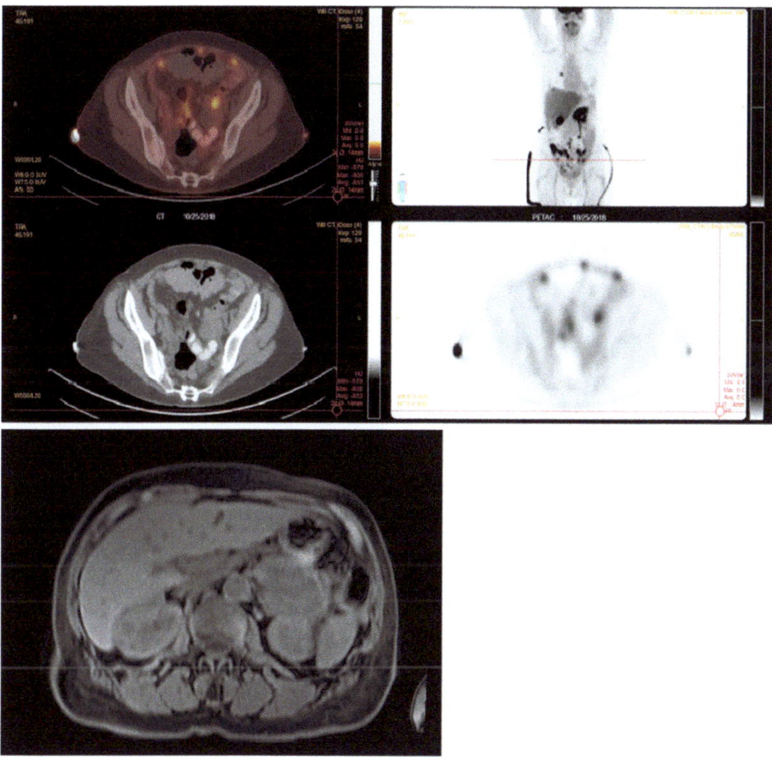

© The Author(s), under exclusive license to Springer Nature Switzerland AG 2022

C. Y. O. Wong, D. Wu, *Phenotypic Oncology PET*,

https://doi.org/10.1007/978-3-031-09737-9_67

67.1   Case 67: Interpretation and Teaching

A1:   F-18 FDG.

A2:   Advanced stage pancreatic cancer with abdominopelvic carcinomatosis.

A3:   Yes. There is focal and asymmetric FDG activity in the right hilar region, suspicious for nodal metastasis.

Teaching Point Pancreatic ductal adenocarcinoma represents majority (90%) of all pancreatic tumors. The only hope for prolonged survival is surgery with complete (R0) resection. Initial imaging by FDG PET has a pivotal role to identify patients who are eligible to curative surgery and those who may benefit of neoadjuvant chemotherapy.

FDG PET/CT detects occult distant metastases not visible on CT performed during initial staging, with limitations of potential low avidity in some primary pancreatic cancers.

FDG PET/CT can evaluate metabolic response after induction treatment for locally advanced pancreatic adenocarcinoma and can serve as a tool to assist the surgical decision.

Reference

Wartski M, Sauvanetb A. 18F-FDG PET/CT in pancreatic adenocarcinoma: a role at initial imaging staging? Diagn Interv Imaging. 2019;100:735–41.

Chapter 68
Case 68: Metabolic Phenotypes in Breast Cancer Bone Metastasis

A: Baseline PET-CT was performed for initial staging right breast cancer. (1) What is the tracer? (2) What does the bone marrow show?

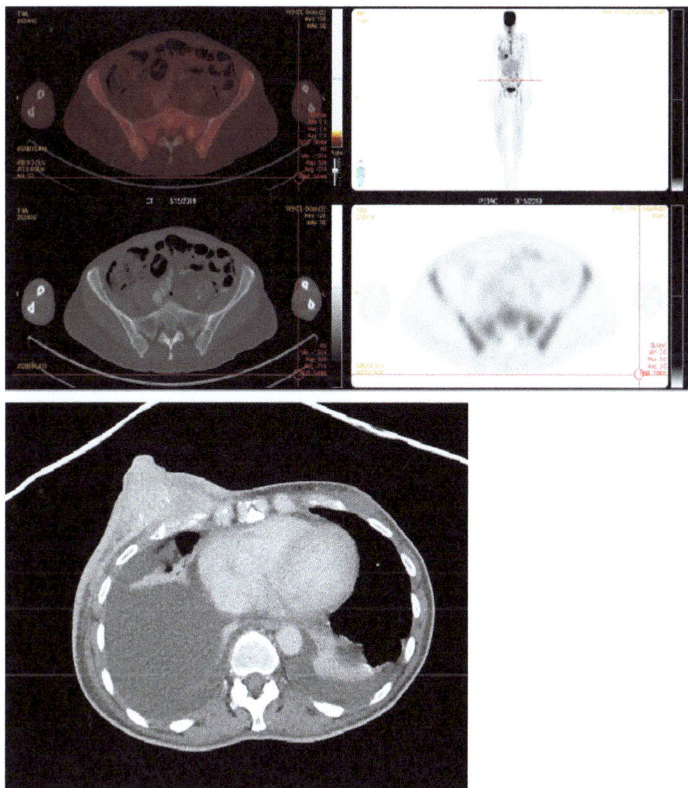

C. Y. O. Wong, D. Wu, *Phenotypic Oncology PET*,
https://doi.org/10.1007/978-3-031-09737-9_68

68.1   Case 68: Interpretation and Teaching

A1:   F-18 FDG.

A2:   The marrow shows diffuse uptake which may be paraneoplastic, hemato-logic, or diffuse infiltrative neoplastic process. It should be correlated with CBC. Without focal avid, lytic, or osteoblastic lesions on the bone, the ulti-mate diagnosis relies on bone marrow biopsy.

Teaching Point PET-CT is more sensitive and more specific than contrast-enhancement CT or bone scan in detecting lytic or mixed bone metastases, or bone marrow involvement. It detects about 50% more lesions than bone scintigraphy.

FDG uptake is more variable in osteoblastic metastases, and it shows less metas-tases than bone scintigraphy.

Higher SUV are observed for osteolytic lesions compared to osteoblastic lesions (mean: 6.77 vs. 0.95). Survival is lower in patients with osteolytic disease compared to others. Also, osteoblastic lesions with no FDG uptake had a better prognosis.

Effective treatment results in bone sclerosis without FDG avidity. The complete healing occurs when such a non-avid sclerotic lesion shows no uptake in bone scan.

Reference

Groheux D, Hindie E. Breast cancer: initial workup and staging with FDG PET/CT. Clinical and Translational Imaging. 2021;9(3):221–31. https://doi.org/10.1007/s40336-021-00426-z.

Chapter 69
Case 69: Concurrent Lung and Pelvic Cancer Phenotypes

A: Baseline PET-CT was performed for diagnosis of lung nodule. (1) What is the tracer? (2) Is the uptake on the nodule significant?

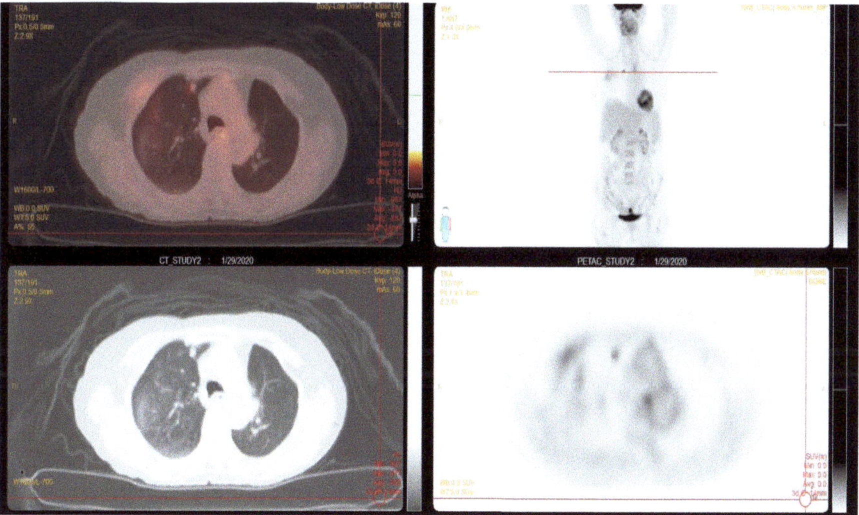

C. Y. O. Wong, D. Wu, *Phenotypic Oncology PET*,
https://doi.org/10.1007/978-3-031-09737-9_69

B: Sagittal images. (1) What is the likely etiology of the avid focus in the pelvis? (2) Is the FDG-avid lung nodule related to this diagnosis? (3) Is there marrow augmentation?

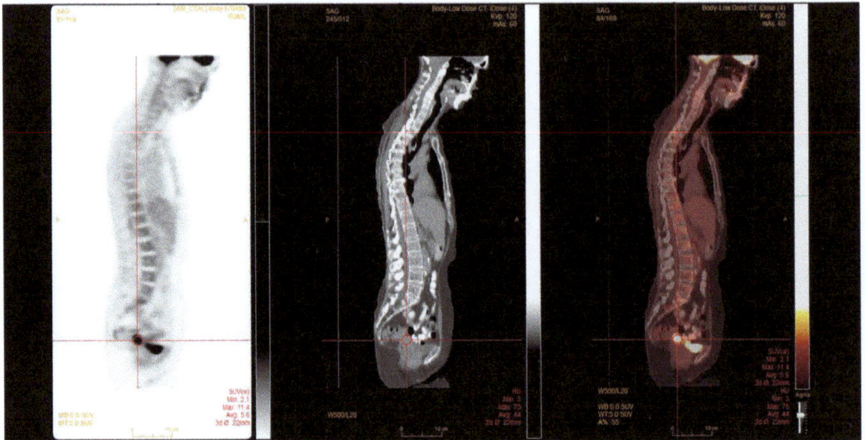

69.1 Case 69: Interpretation and Teaching

A1:   F-18 FDG.

A2:   Yes, any focal uptake in a pulmonary nodule irrespective of degree is likely significant to suspect malignancy.

B1:   It is likely endocervical cancer with intense FDG avidity.

B2:   Since the lung nodule has mild FDG avidity, it is likely a different metabolic phenotype pointing to a low-grade primary lung adenocarcinoma, while the endocervical cancer has a high metabolism which is likely from squamous cell carcinoma.

B3:   The marrow shows diffuse uptake which may be paraneoplastic, hematologic, or diffuse infiltrative neoplastic process. It should be correlated with CBC. Without focal avid, lytic, or osteoblastic lesions on the bone, the ultimate diagnosis relies on the marrow biopsy.

Teaching Point It is quite common to detect two malignancies in the single PET scan. Not all avid foci are the same from clonal point of view. Thus, recognition of different metabolic phenotypes is important by not overcalling the cancer to the advanced stage. In this case, it is likely the lung and cervical cancer, with each one of the two cancers in its early stage.

Higher primary tumor FDG uptake predicts higher nodal and distant metastatic potential in cervical cancer patients. Double SUV will double the chance of metastasis. Patients with higher SUV in cervical tumor may need a close follow-up by PET-CT.

Reference

Yilmaz M, Mustafa Adli M, Celen Z, et al. FDG PET-CT in cervical cancer: relationship between primary tumor FDG uptake and metastatic potential. Nucl Med Commun. 2010;31(6):526–31.

Chapter 70
Case 70: Inflammatory Breast Cancer (IBC)

A: PET-CT and whole-body bone scan staging of biopsy-proven right breast cancer. (1) What are the tracers for both imaging sets? (2) Are there any bone lesions? (3) What other imaging is needed?

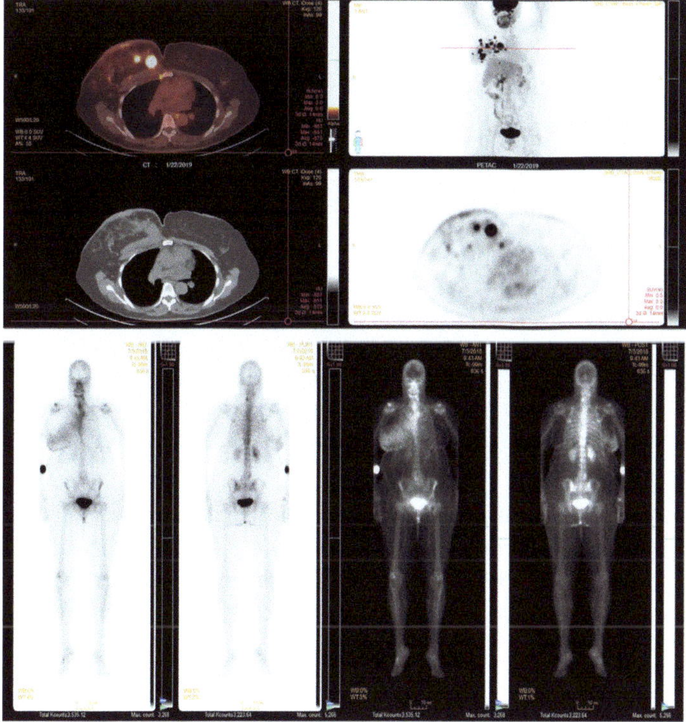

C. Y. O. Wong, D. Wu, *Phenotypic Oncology PET*, https://doi.org/10.1007/978-3-031-09737-9_70

70.1 Case 70: Interpretation and Teaching

A1: F-18 FDG and Tc-99 m MDP (F-18 NaF PET scan offers a high-resolution scan; the bone scan using single photon of F-18 NaF was initially performed in early history of nuclear medicine before Tc-99 m MDP became widely available).

A2: Degenerative changes without avid lesions in both PET and bone scans. The avid lesion by right parasternal area is most likely nodal metastasis in right internal mammary region.

A3: MRI is most likely for full evaluation of breasts and any brachial plexus involvement. CT is limited in this aspect of evaluation.

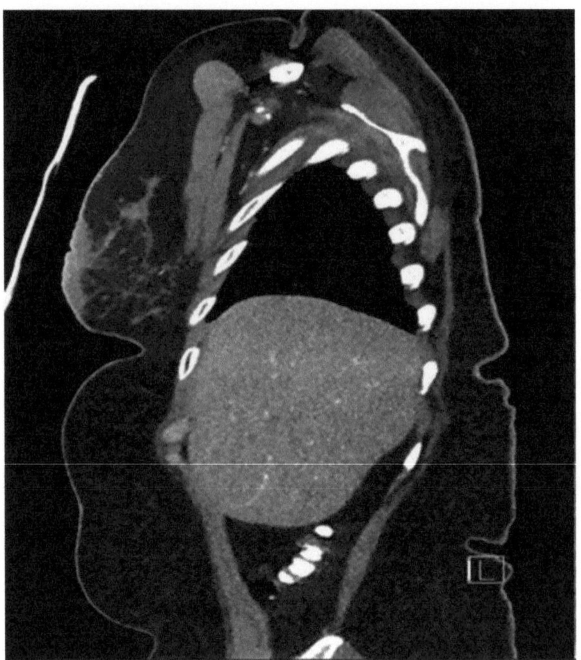

Teaching Point Over ¾ of the patients with inflammatory breast cancer (IBC) present with axillary lymph node involvement and about 40% with distant metastases. F-18 FDG PET/CT detects additional locoregional lymph node metastases and distant metastases in about 10% of patients that were not detected with standard conventional imaging modalities.

Reference

van Uden DJP, Prins MW, Siesling S, et al. [18F]FDG PET/CT in the staging of inflammatory breast cancer: a systematic review. Crit Rev. Oncol Hematol. 2020;151:102943. https://doi.org/10.1016/j.critrevonc.2020.102943.

Chapter 71
Case 71: Recurrent High-Grade Urothelial Carcinoma

A: Patient is a 64-year-old male with history of high-grade urothelial carcinoma of bladder trigone base, status post-transurethral resection and completed chemotherapy nearly 2 years ago. Restaging PET-CT was requested due to gross hematuria and concerns for recurrent disease. (1) What is the tracer? (2) Is there any evidence for recurrent disease? (3) Is there PET-CT finding suggestive of right peri-vesical involvement? (4) What happened to the right kidney and ureter?

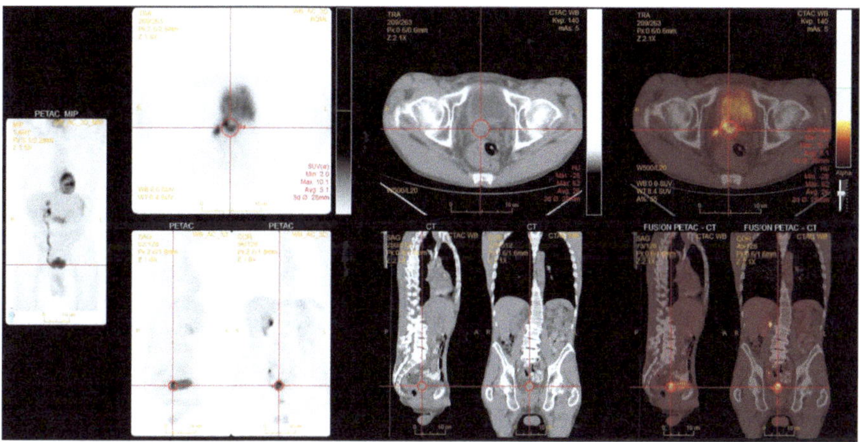

227

C. Y. O. Wong, D. Wu, *Phenotypic Oncology PET*,
https://doi.org/10.1007/978-3-031-09737-9_71

71.1   Case 71: Interpretation and Teaching

A1:   F-18 FDG.

A2:   Yes. The CT shows thickened bladder wall in the right trigone compared to the contralateral, suspicious for recurrent urothelial carcinoma.

A3:   Posterior to the focal thickened right trigone bladder wall, there is fullness with heterogeneous FDG intensity higher than the urine FDG activity, suspicious for peri-vesical tumor invasion macroscopically, indicating stage III disease.

A4:   Intense urine FDG activity is seen in the dilated right renal collecting system and renal pelvis as well as within the tortuous and dilated right ureter, indicating obstructive right hydroureteronephrosis, likely secondary to recurrent tumor involving the right trigone bladder wall leading to high-grade obstruction of the right ureter orifice.

Teaching Point High-grade urothelial carcinoma is an aggressive malignant tumor with a high rate of recurrence, progression, and cancer-specific mortality. After initial successful treatment, there are approximately 40% rate of recurrence and 20% rate of progression at 5 years. This case reveals recurrent tumor involving the right trigone bladder wall and disease progression with invasion into peri-vesical tissue at 2 years. The finding of obstructive right hydronephrosis and hydroureter is not only an indirect evidence of recurrent bladder cancer but also an indication of the urgency for urological intervention to prevent permanent kidney damage.

References

Magers MJ, Lopez-Beltran A, Montironi R, et al. Staging of bladder cancer. Histopathology. 2019;74(1):112–34.

Reisz PA, Laviana AA, Chang SS. Management of high-grade T1 urothelial carcinoma. Curr Urol Rep. 2018;19:103.

Chapter 72
Case 72: Primary Thyroid Lymphoma (PTL)

A: Initial staging PET-CT was performed in a 51-year-old female with newly diagnosed extra-nodal marginal zone lymphoma of right thyroid, initially via FNA cytology and then confirmed with right thyroid incisional biopsy. Pertinent medical history is significant for Hashimoto's autoimmune thyroiditis. (1) What is the tracer? (2) Is the biopsy-proven lymphoma involving one side or bilateral thyroid gland? (3) There are two or three small foci of mild to moderate FDG activity in the mediastinum. Are they representing additional lymphomas?

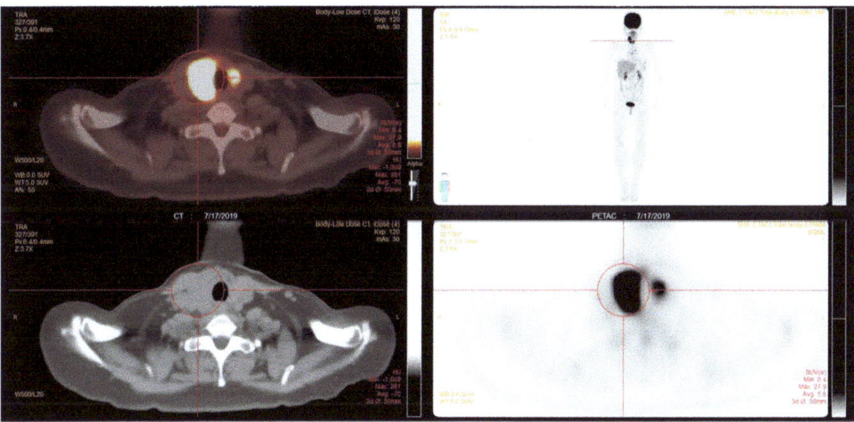

C. Y. O. Wong, D. Wu, *Phenotypic Oncology PET*,
https://doi.org/10.1007/978-3-031-09737-9_72

B: After completion of chemoradiation, two restaging PET-CT studies were performed as the following, with time interval of 4 months and 23 months from the initial PET-CT, respectively. (1) How was the treatment response of the PTL? What is the Lugano score? (2) What is the interpretation of the mediastinal FDG activities? (3) What's the likely cause of the new right axillary adenopathy?

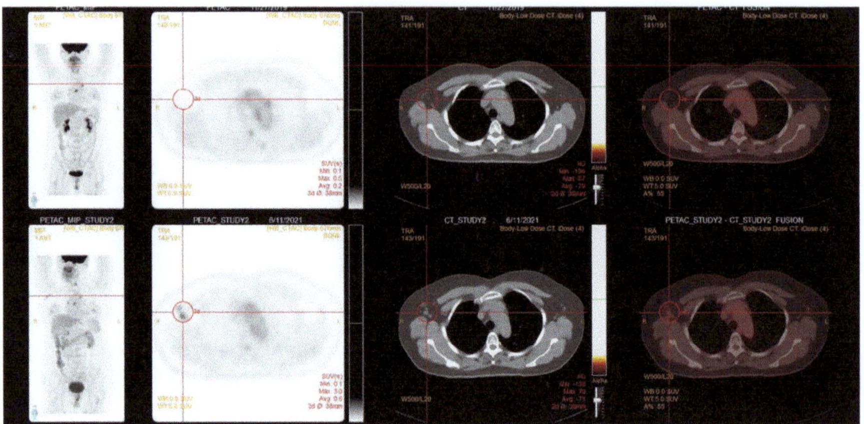

72.1 Case 72: Interpretation and Teaching

A1: F-18 FDG.

A2: The primary thyroid lymphoma (PTL) involves bilateral thyroid lobes, right great than left, in variable sizes and FDG intensities.

A3: The foci of FDG activity scattered in the bilateral pre-vascular and subcarinal mediastinum have a mild to moderate intensity, likely unrelated to lymphoma, although it cannot be ruled out. Attention on follow-up imaging is recommended.

B1: The treatment response to chemoradiation is excellent, with a Lugano score of 1–2, as FDG activity in the thyroid region is below the mediastinal blood pool.

B2: In contrast, the foci of FDG activity in the mediastinum remain, with essentially stable intensities, providing further evidence for a non-lymphoma etiology, such as granulomatous disease or reactive changes.

B3: The new finding of FDG-avid adenopathy in the right axillary region is most likely due to reactive changes to vaccination during the COVID-19 pandemic. Clinical correlation suggests the likely cause.

Teaching Point Primary thyroid lymphoma (PTL) is a rare primary thyroid malignancy, characterized by lymphomatous involving the thyroid gland only, without contiguous spread or distant involvement of other organs or tissues, as shown in this case. PTL is usually manifested by a rapidly growing and painless thyroid masses in patients with a history of Hashimoto's thyroiditis. Surgical resection used to be the mainstay of treatment. However, combined chemoradiation is increasingly utilized as the first line of therapy, often with a favorable and sustainable response.

References

Graff-Baker A, Roman SA, Thomas DC, Udelsman R, Sosa JA. Prognosis of primary thyroid lymphoma: demographic, clinical, and pathologic predictors of survival in 1,408 cases. Surgery. 2009;146(6):1105–15.

Pavlidis ET, Pavlidis TE. A review of primary thyroid lymphoma: molecular factors, diagnosis and management. J Investig Surg. 2019;32(2):137–42.

Stein SA, Wartofsky L. Primary thyroid lymphoma: a clinical review. J Clin Endocrinol Metab. 2013;98(8):3131–18.

Chapter 73
Case 73: High-Grade Tonsil Large B-Cell Lymphoma

A: Initial PET-CT was performed in a 48-year-old female with newly diagnosed high-grade large B-cell lymphoma of left tonsil. Immunohistochemistry (IHC) positive for CD10, CD20, CD79A, BCL-6, and focal BCL-2, Ki-67 > 95%. (1) What is the tracer? (2) Is there any evidence for misregistration of PET and CT? (3) Did lymphoma involve the right tonsil?

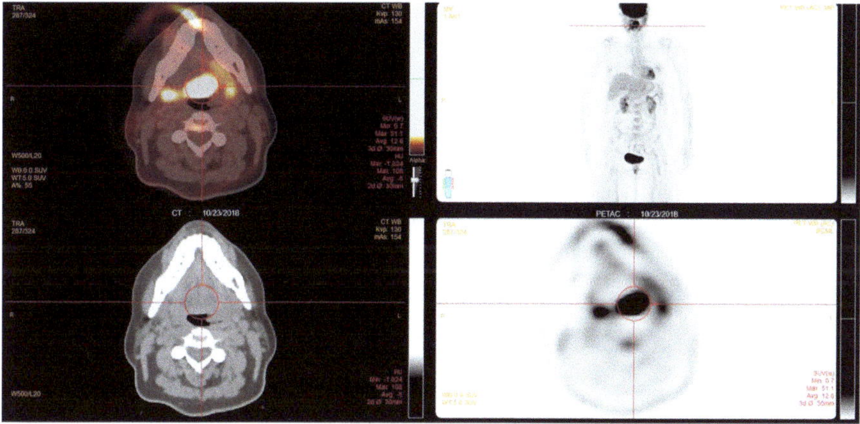

C. Y. O. Wong, D. Wu, *Phenotypic Oncology PET*, https://doi.org/10.1007/978-3-031-09737-9_73

B: Patient received R-CHOP × 3 cycles followed by consolidative radiation. Restaging PET-CT was performed with selected image as the following: (1) How was the response to chemoradiation? (2) What's Lugano score? (3) Based on the IHC, what do we recommend in terms of imaging follow-up?

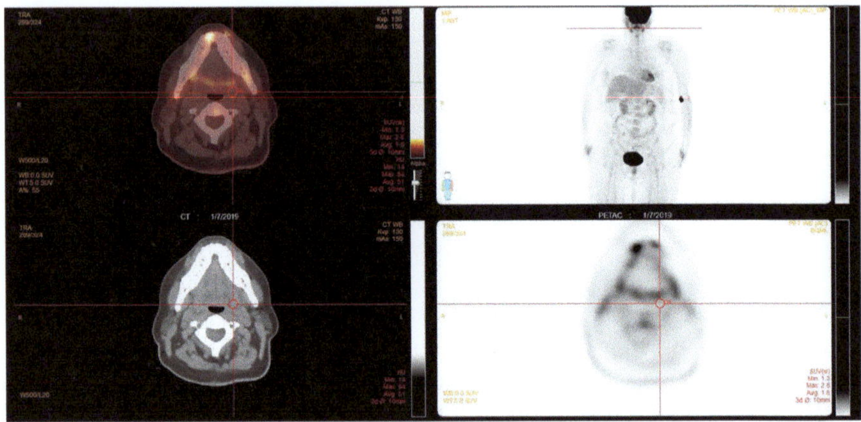

73.1   Case 73: Interpretation and Teaching

A1:   F-18 FDG.

A2:   Yes, there is visual misregistration between the PET and CT images, especially the head and neck region, best appreciated on the PET-CT axial fusion image.

A3:   Yes. Despite the misregistration, there is an FDG-avid left tonsillar mass with max SUV 54.7, consistent with biopsy-proven left tonsil high-grade large B-cell lymphoma. CT imaging of the right tonsil is unremarkable; however, there is focal and moderate FDG activity, max SUV 10.8, suspicious for lymphomatous involvement of the Waldeyer's ring including right tonsil.

B1:   The response to chemoradiation is excellent.

B2:   There is no discrete appreciable FDG activity in the Waldeyer's ring, with a special reference to the left tonsillar region, consistent with Lugano score 1.

B3:   The patient achieved complete remission based on FDG PET criteria; however, close imaging follow-up is recommended, given the IHC evidence of triple expression and high rate of proliferation.

Teaching Point Primary tonsil lymphoma or primary lymphoma of Waldeyer's ring is an extranodal but not an extra-lymphatic malignant lymphoma, often involving the lymphoid tissues of the tonsils, the nasopharynx, and base of the tongue. PTLs typically have favorable outcomes/prognosis after standard chemoradiation, as majority (about 80%) of the primary tonsil or Waldeyer's ring lymphomas present as localized disease (i.e., stage IE or IIE). However, there is IHC evidence of triple expression in this patient's high-grade lymphoma. Thus, close imaging follow-up shall be recommended or at the discretion of the referring physician.

References

Mohammadianpanah M, Daneshbod Y, Ramzi M, et al. Primary tonsillar lymphomas according to the new world health organization classification: to report 87 cases and literature review and analysis. Ann Hematol. 2010;89(10):993–1001.

Saul SH, Kapadia SB. Primary lymphoma of Waldeyer's ring. Clinicopathologic study of 68 cases. Cancer. 1985;56(1):157–66.

Chapter 74
Case 74: Phenotypic Pattern of Primary Renal DLBCL with Double Expressor

A: Patient is an 87-year-old female with newly diagnosed primary left renal lymphoma, consistent with diffuse large B-cell lymphoma, with high proliferative rate and double expressor. PET-CT was performed for initial staging. (1) What is the tracer? (2) Is there any evidence of extrarenal malignant involvement?

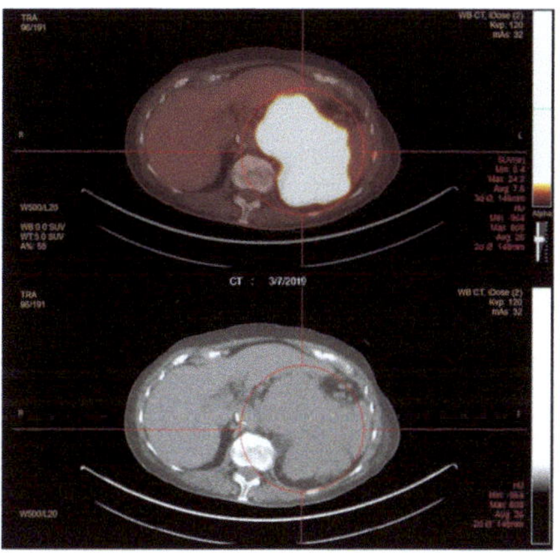 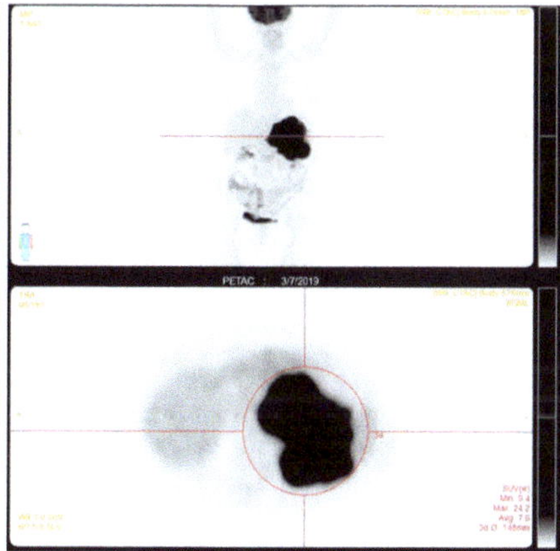

C. Y. O. Wong, D. Wu, *Phenotypic Oncology PET*,
https://doi.org/10.1007/978-3-031-09737-9_74

B: Serial restaging PET-CTs were performed during and after completion of chemotherapy and radiation. (1) How was the response? (2) What's the appropriate recommendation?

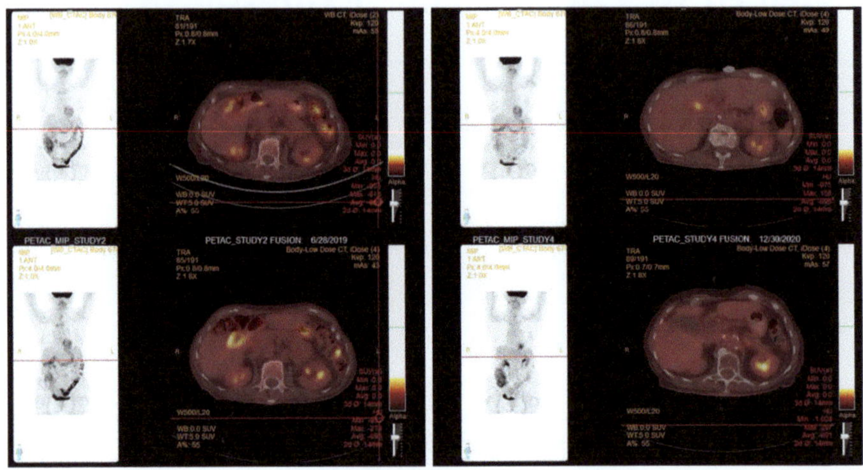

74.1 Case 74: Interpretation and Teaching

A1:   F-18 FDG.

A2:   No. Images show a large irregular left renal mass with intense FDG activity, consistent with biopsy-proven left renal diffuse large B-cell lymphoma.

B1:   The response to chemotherapy is favorable, and several restaging PET-CT studies show no discrete abnormal FDG activity in the left kidney in comparison to the right kidney, consistent with Lugano score 1.

B2:   Despite the favorable response and complete remission achieved, follow-up PET-CT is recommended, due to the pathological features of high proliferative rate and double expressor.

Teaching Point Double-expressor lymphoma (DEL) is pathologically defined as overexpression of MYC and BCL2 proteins not related to underlying chromosomal rearrangements. The prognosis of patients with DEL is very poor. The 5-year overall survival (OS) is only approximately 40% with R-CHOP (rituximab, cyclophosphamide, doxorubicin, vincristine, and prednisone). Given the poor outcomes after standard chemotherapy, close imaging follow-up with or without additional treatment is imperative to detect relapsed or recurrent disease.

References

Bokhari SRA, Inayat F, Bokhari MR, et al. Primary renal lymphoma: a comprehensive review of the pathophysiology, clinical presentation, imaging features, management and prognosis. BMJ Case Rep. 2020;13(6):e235076.

Taneja A, Kumar V, Chandra AB. Primary renal lymphoma: a population-based analysis using the SEER program (1973-2015). Eur J Haematol. 2020;1104(5):390–9.

Chapter 75
Case 75: Recurrent Primary Colonic Lymphoma (PCL)

A: Diagnostic PET-CT was performed in a 68-year-old male with biopsy findings of atypical lymphoid infiltrate, suspicious for lymphoma in the ascending colon 2 weeks ago. (1) What's the tracer? (2) What's the PET-CT impression, given the nonconclusive pathology? (3) Is there any evidence of extra-colonic involvement?

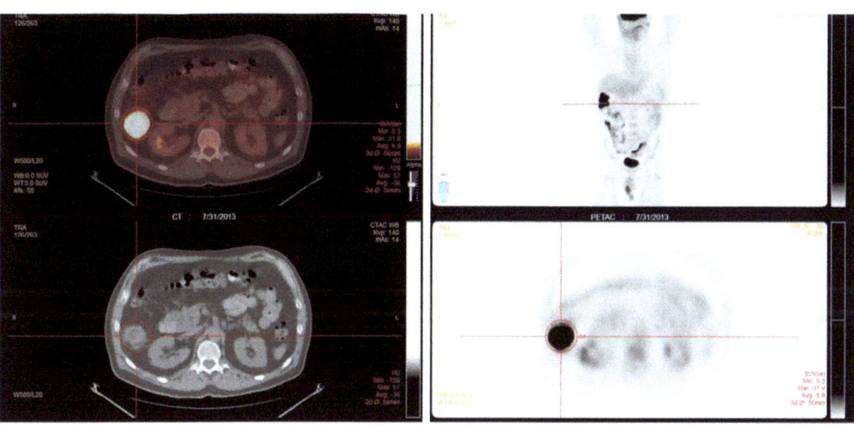

C. Y. O. Wong, D. Wu, *Phenotypic Oncology PET*, https://doi.org/10.1007/978-3-031-09737-9_75

B: Seven years after successful treatment including segmental colectomy and chemotherapy, a new biopsy of right colon was positive for recurrent DLBCL, for which first restaging PET-CT was performed (upper panel). The bottom panel is second restaging PET-CT following right colectomy including ileocolic anastomosis and chemotherapy. (1) Is the recurrent lymphoma metabolically similar or different from the original lymphoma? (2) How was the response to new treatment and what's Lugano score?

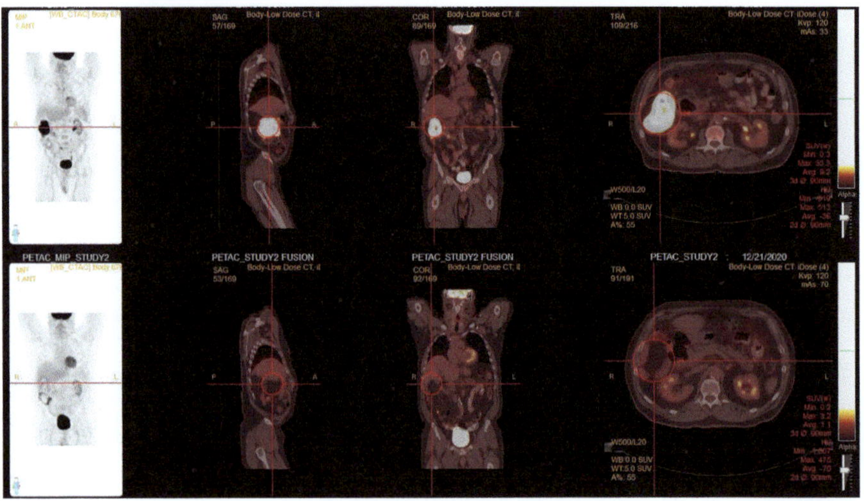

75.1   Case 75: Interpretation and Teaching

A1:   F-18 FDG.

A2:   PET-CT shows a large ascending colon mass near the hepatic flexure with intense FDG uptake, max SUV 31.9, highly suggestive of malignant lymphoma.

A3:   Imaging of the remainder of the abdomen, pelvis, chest, or the visualized portion of the head and neck is unremarkable, without extra-colonic involvement. The findings are consistent with primary colonic lymphoma (PCL).

B1:   The biopsy-proven recurrent ascending colon DLBCL is very similar to the prior disease in terms of metabolic activity, with current max SUV 33.3 in comparison to the prior max SUV 31.9 7 years ago.

B2:   The response is excellent, without discrete appreciable FDG activity at the recurrent disease site. Of note, nonspecific FDG activities are noted in the right lower quadrant, likely due to postsurgical changes rather than lymphomatous activity. Therefore, the findings are consistent with Lugano score 1×

Teaching Point Primary colonic lymphoma (PCL) is a rare disease accounting for less than 1% of large bowel malignancy. The most common location of PCL is the cecum (60%), followed by the ascending colon (27%) and the sigmoid colon (13%). This case shows primary and recurrent PCL involving the ascending colon near the hepatic flexure, with a favorable response to combined surgical resection and chemotherapy.

References

Doolabh N, Anthony T, Simmang C, et al. Primary colonic lymphoma. J Surg Oncol. 2000;74(4):257–62.

Gonzales QH, Heslin MJ, Davila-Cervantes A, et al. Primary colonic lymphoma. Am Surg. 2008;74(3):214–6.

Chapter 76
Case 76: Maxillofacial Extranodal Marginal Zone Malignant B-Cell Lymphoma

A: Patient is an 88-year-old male with diagnostic CT showing a lobulated subcutaneous mass centered within the left nasolabial fold, with mottled appearance of the left maxilla medial wall and involving the hard palate. MR imaging revealed a vertical elongated left subcutaneous enhancing soft tissue mass of 7.9 cm overlying the left nasal bone and nasal bridge, with involvement of the left hard palate. Subsequent biopsy was positive for marginal zone malignant B-cell lymphoma of left maxillofacial. PET-CT was performed for initial staging. (1) What is the tracer? (2) Is there any evidence of lymphomatous involvement of the brain base? (3) Any imaging evidence of bone marrow involvement?

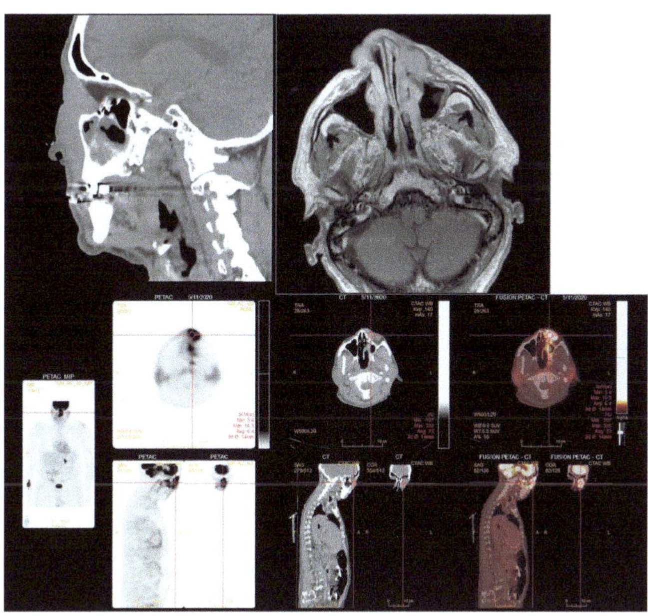

© The Author(s), under exclusive license to Springer Nature Switzerland AG 2022

C. Y. O. Wong, D. Wu, *Phenotypic Oncology PET*, https://doi.org/10.1007/978-3-031-09737-9_76

76.1   Case 76: Interpretation and Teaching

A1:   F-18 FDG.

A2:   No. The MIP and sagittal PET-CT images, in conjunction with MR imaging, show no abnormal FDG activity to suggest malignant involvement of the brain base, especially the ethmoidal sinuses or the sphenoidal sinuses.

A3:   Minimal FDG activity is noted in the left shoulder region likely due to arthritic/degenerative changes. FDG infiltration is noted in the right wrist injection site/IV line. But there is no discrete focal abnormal FDG activity to suggestive bone marrow involvement. Nevertheless, due to the rarity of maxillofacial malignant lymphoma, bone marrow biopsy was performed for further restaging; it returned positive for B-cell lymphoma involving approximately 30% of marrow cellularity.

Teaching Point Maxillofacial lymphoma is an extremely rare extranodal malignancy. FDG PET-CT shows no evidence of any nodal involvement above and below the diaphragm; however, it failed to reveal any bone marrow involvement, which is false negative given the positive BM biopsy, indicating that a negative FDG PET-CT cannot exclude the possibility of bone marrow involvement. In contrast, focally avid marrow lesions suggesting lymphoma render marrow biopsy unnecessary.

References

MacDonald D, Li T, Leung SF, et al. Extranodal lymphoma arising within the maxillary alveolus: a case report. Oral Surg Oral Med Oral Pathol Oral Radiol. 2017;124(3):e233–8.

MacDonald D, Martin M, Savage K. Maxillofacial lymphomas. Br J Radiol. 2021;94(1120): 20191041.

Chapter 77
Case 77: Primary Dural Lymphoma (PDL) with Leptomeningeal and Scalp Involvement

A: Initial PET-CT in a 67-year-old female with newly diagnosed DLBCL via a biopsy of left anterior superior orbital lesion. Recent MRI revealed diffuse thickening of the leptomeninges along the left cerebral convexity (data not shown). Cerebrospinal fluid (CSF) cytology showed atypical lymphoid cells suspicious for lymphoma, while marrow biopsy was negative. (1) What is the tracer? (2) Is there any evidence of scalp/subcutaneous involvement? (3) Is there any evidence of primary cerebral involvement?

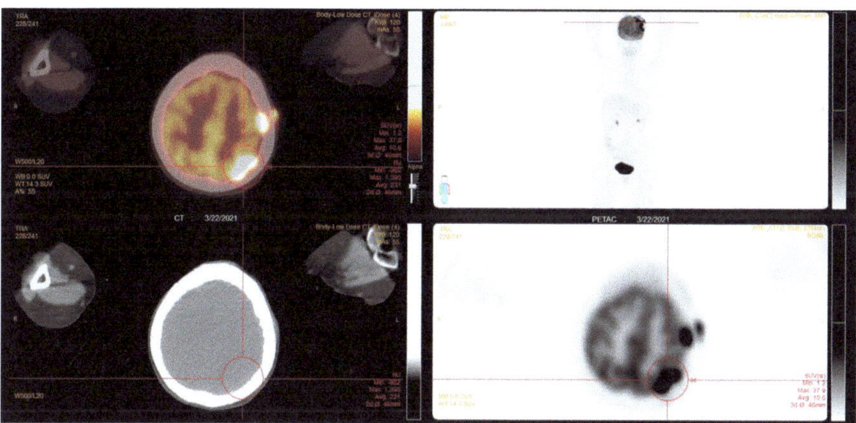

C. Y. O. Wong, D. Wu, *Phenotypic Oncology PET*,
https://doi.org/10.1007/978-3-031-09737-9_77

B: Restaging PET-CT during and after completion of chemotherapy, including hospital admission for administration of high-dose methotrexate (MTX) and monitoring for MTX levels and electrolytes in addition to conventional R-CHOP for a total of six cycles. (1) How was treatment response? (2) What's the Lugano score?

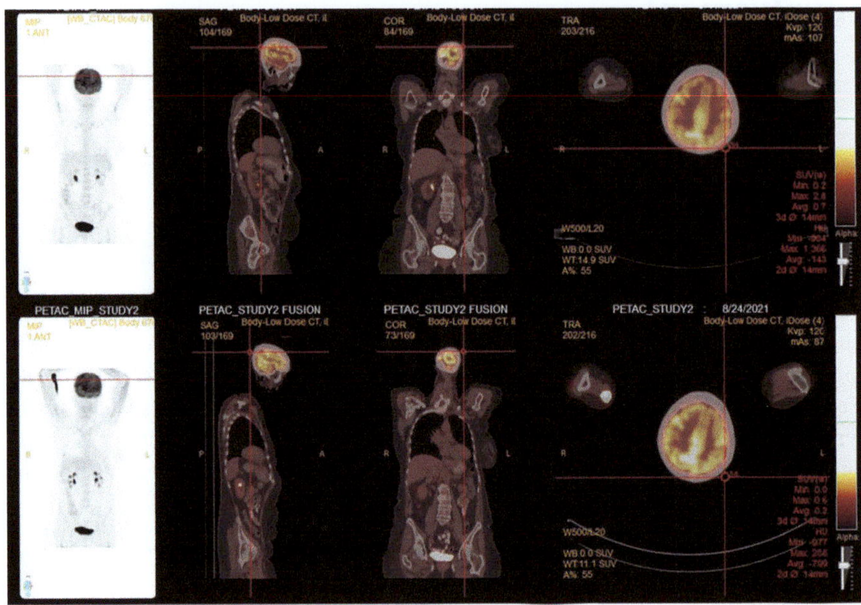

77.1 Case 77: Interpretation and Teaching

A1: F-18 FDG.

A2: Yes. There is a focal and moderate FDG activity in the left anterolateral scalp/ subcutaneous region, likely the biopsy site for DLBCL. Adjacent to this lesion, there is a focus of intense FDG activity corresponding to the dura/ meninges, indicating primary dural lymphoma (PDL) with direct invasion/ penetration into overlying skull and scalp. Otherwise, there is no evidence of lymphomatous involvement in the peripheral tissue.

A3: No, there is no evidence of primary cerebral involvement on MR imaging (data not shown) or FDG PET-CT.

B1: The response to R-CHOP plus high dose of MTX was excellent.

B2: Lugano score was 1 for both interim and end-chemotherapy PET-CT in that there is no appreciable FDG activity over background level.

Teaching Point Primary dural lymphoma (PDL) is a rare variant of primary central nervous system (CNS) lymphoma (see details about PCNSL in Case 78). Radiologically, PDL can be misdiagnosed as meningioma, due to its dura mater origin. As shown in this case, direct invasion/penetration of the overlying skull/ scalp can happen, but there is no systemic or peripheral involvement. Although CNS cytology examination was positive for atypical lymphoid cells, likely due to shedding, there is no involvement of the primary brain parenchyma, indicating that intrathecal chemotherapy may be avoided without affecting the treatment efficiency. Indeed, this patient received in-hospital high dose of MTX with close monitoring of MTX levels and electrolytes, with an excellent response, and achieved complete remission based on FDG PET-CT criteria.

Reference

Karschnia P, Batchelor TT, Jordan JT, et al. Primary dural lymphomas: clinical presentation, management, and outcome. Cancer. 2020;126(12):2811–20.

Chapter 78
Case 78: Primary CNS Lymphoma (PCNSL)

A: Patient is a 72-year-old male with newly diagnosed DLBCL via biopsy of right frontal brain lesion 2 weeks ago. Patient denied prior history of lymphoma. (1) What is the tracer? (2) What do the low-density changes on MRI and hypometabolism on PET in the adjacent brain parenchyma represent? (3) Is there any evidence of systemic lymphomatous involvement? (4) How is the prognosis?

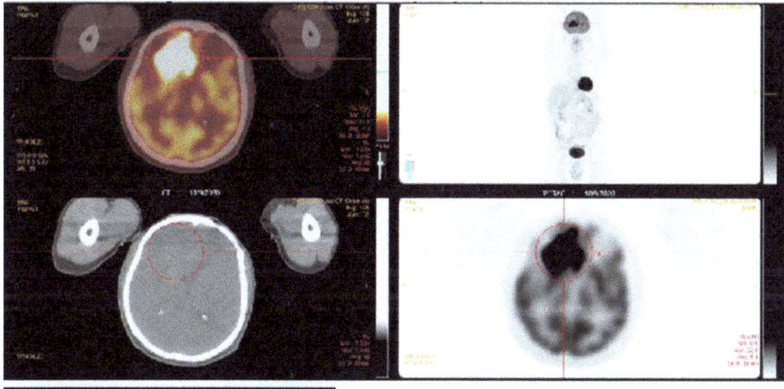

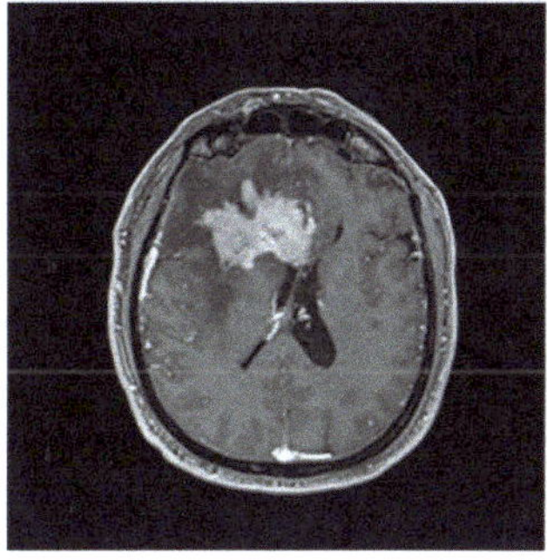

C. Y. O. Wong, D. Wu, *Phenotypic Oncology PET*,
https://doi.org/10.1007/978-3-031-09737-9_78

78.1   Case 78: Interpretation and Teaching

A1:   F-18 FDG.

A2:   The low-density changes on MR imaging and hypometabolism on FDG PET are typical for vasogenic edema secondary to mass effects, which can be seen in any primary or metastatic brain tumors.

A3:   No, there is no evidence for peripheral involvement in the head/neck, chest, abdomen, pelvis, or the visualized extremities.

A4:   The prognosis is very poor. Despite timely treatment with systemic and intra-thecal chemotherapy, the patient passed away due to decline in performance, contraction of COVID-19 pneumonia, and multiple organ failure 3 months later.

Teaching Point Primary CNS lymphoma (PCNSL) is a rare form of malignant lymphoma that typically confines to the brain parenchyma as shown in this case. Additional involvements include the spinal cord, the eyes, and the cerebrospinal fluid (CSF). The primary dural lymphoma (PDL) is generally considered as a rare variant of PCNSL (see details about PDL in Case 77). PCNSL is different from secondary CNS lymphoma (SCNSL, in Case 59), due to a lack of history of systemic lymphoma and no current evidence of lymphomatous involvement in the peripheral tissue. The prognosis of PCNSL is very poor, in part due to blood-brain barrier (BBB) that reduces the efficiency of systemic and/or intrathecal chemotherapies.

References

Grommes C, Rubenstein JL, DeAngelis LM, et al. Comprehensive approach to diagnosis and treatment of newly diagnosed primary CNS lymphoma. Neuro-Oncology. 2019;21(3):296–305.

Hoang-Xuan K, Bessell E, Bromberg J, et al. Diagnosis and treatment of primary CNS lymphoma in immunocompetent patients: guidelines from the European Association for Nero-Oncology. Lancet Oncol. 2015;16(7):e322–32.

Chapter 79
Case 79: Primary Gastric Lymphoma (PGL)

A: Initial PET-CT in a 51-year-old female with biopsy-proven large B-cell lymphoma of the stomach. (1) What is the tracer? (2) Is there any evidence of extragastric lymphomatous involvement?

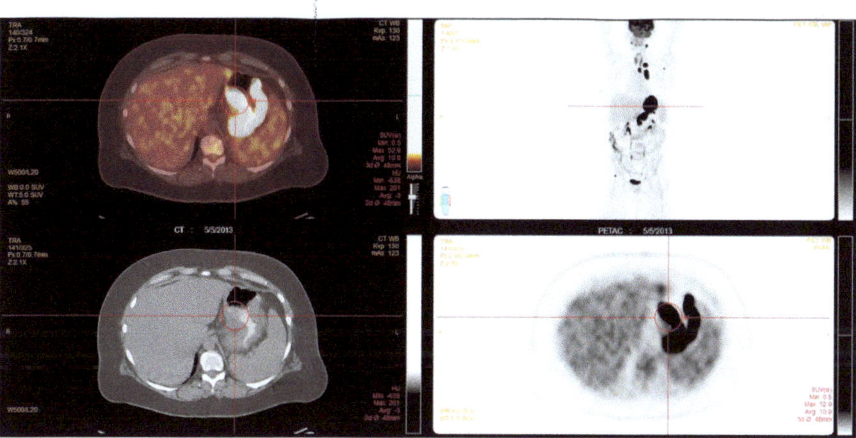

C. Y. O. Wong, D. Wu, *Phenotypic Oncology PET*, https://doi.org/10.1007/978-3-031-09737-9_79

B: Restaging PET-CT scans during and after completion of chemotherapy with R-CHOP showed incidental findings including focal activity in the right axilla without CT correlate (far left) and persistent and increasing tracer activity in the thyroid. (1) How was the response to chemotherapy? (2) What is the Lugano score? (3) What is the likely cause of the right axillary activity? (4) Is the thyroid activity benign or malignant?

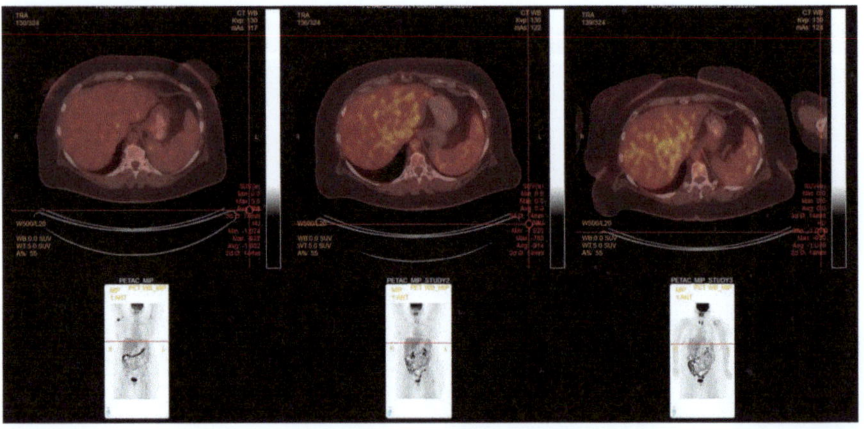

79.1 Case 79: Interpretation and Teaching

A1: F-18 FDG.

A2: Yes. In addition to diffuse involvement of the greater curvature of the stomach and antrum, FDG-avid adenopathy is noted in the bilateral neck, the mediastinum, the left axilla, the peri-gastric region, and the right inguinal area, suspicious for lymphoma above and below the diaphragm.

B1: The response to chemotherapy is excellent, as evidenced by interval resolution of all the FDG-avid lymph nodes above and below the diaphragm. The previously noted diffuse gastric wall thickening has resolved on the concurrent CT, with markedly decreased FDG activity in the gastric wall. Although minimal FDG activity is noted on the mucosa surface, consecutive two gastric biopsies showed mild congestion or chronic inactive gastritis but no evidence of lymphoma.

B2: The Lugano score is 1× (mucosal activity unrelated to lymphoma).

B3: The baseline PET-CT showed no lymphomatous involvement of the right axilla. Therefore, the transient FDG activity without CT correlate is most likely due to an inflammatory process, or secondary to FDG infiltration from right arm injection site.

B4: In retrospect, the thyroid uptake was present on the baseline PET-CT scan. It is persistent with variable but mild to moderate FDG activity. The interval stability and the diffuse pattern are suggestive of a benign etiology.

Teaching Point Primary gastric lymphomas (PGL) are a distinct extra-nodal lymphoproliferative disease with two main histological types: DLBCL and mucosa-associated lymphoid tissue (MALT). The gastric body and antrum are the most commonly involving sites as shown in this case. In contrast to DLBCL, gastric MALT lymphoma is a low-grade B-cell lymphoma, and most cases (about 90%) are directly related to *H. pylori* infection. Review of literature shows chemotherapy with R-CHOP leading to a better outcome in comparison to patients received CHOP, with an overall good prognosis.

References

Diamantidis MD, Papaioannou M, Hatjiharissi E. Primary gastric non-Hodgkin lymphomas: recent advances regarding disease pathogenesis and treatment. World J Gastroenterol. 2021;27(35):5932–45.

Roukos DH, Hottenrott C, Encke A, et al. Primary gastric lymphoma: a clinicopathologic study with literature review. Surg Oncol. 1994;3(2):115–25.

Chapter 80
Case 80: Residual Primary Prostate Lymphoma (PPL)

A: Patient is a 52-year-old male with history of benign prostate hyperplasia (BPH) undergoing transurethral resection. Pathology returned positive for diffuse large B-cell lymphoma (DLBCL). PET-CT was performed for staging. (1) What is the tracer? (2) What's PET-CT impression about the prostate bed? (3) There is focal tracer activity in the cecal region without definite CT correlate. What's the recommendation?

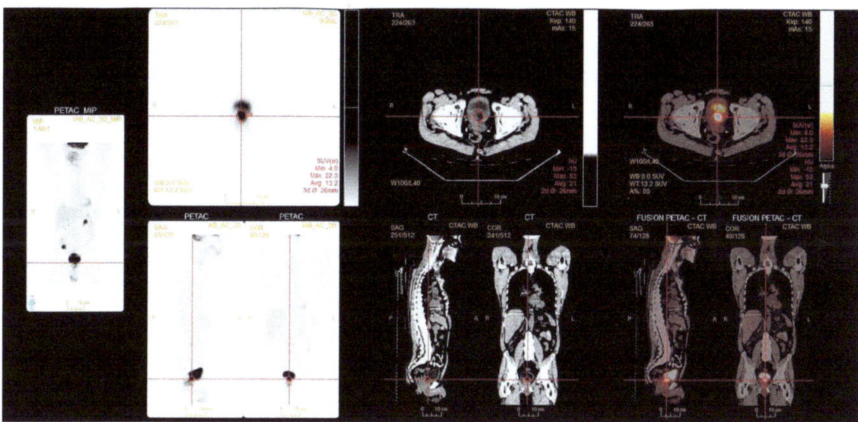

C. Y. O. Wong, D. Wu, *Phenotypic Oncology PET*, https://doi.org/10.1007/978-3-031-09737-9_80

B: Patient underwent cecum biopsy showing tubulovillous adenoma with high-grade dysplasia, followed by segmental ileocolectomy confirming the presence of adenoma but no evidence of malignancy. Two restaging PET-CT scans were performed after completion of six cycles of R-CHOP followed by consolidative radiation therapy. (1) How was the response of PPL to therapies and what's Lugano score? (2) What is the likely cause of the bone marrow uptake (lower panel dated May 11, 2015)?

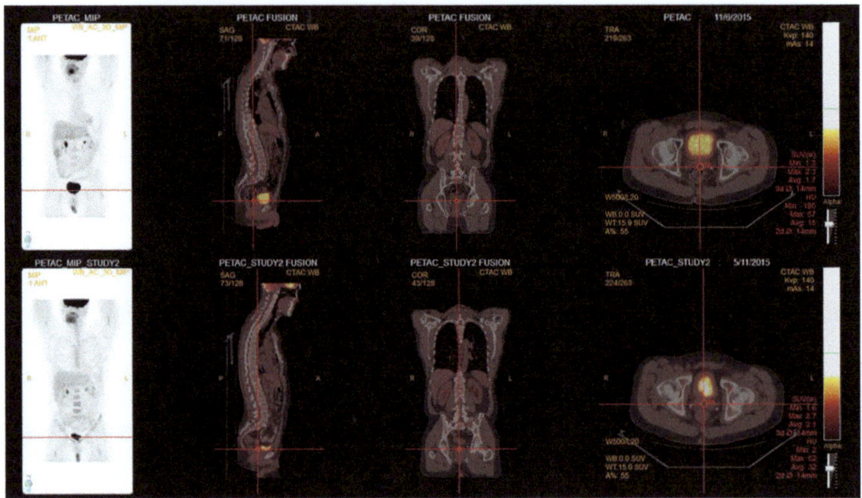

80.1 Case 80: Interpretation and Teaching

A1: F-18 FDG.

A2: Postsurgical changes are noted in the central portion of the prostate bed. FDG-avid soft tissues are noted in the surrounding, with tracer intensity higher than the urinary activity, max SUV 22.3, highly suggestive of residual DLBCL.

A3: The focal FDG activity in cecal region without CT correlate may represent a benign etiology, but colonic primary malignancy or lymphomatous involvement cannot be excluded. Therefore, further workup such as colonoscopy with biopsy if needed shall be recommended.

B1: The response to therapies is favorable, without appreciable FDG activity in the prostate bed for two consecutive scans in a row, consistent with Lugano score 1.

B2: The first restaging study (the lower panel dated May 11, 2015) was performed approximately 1 month following completion of R-CHOP. The mild and diffuse bone marrow FDG activity is most likely due to residual reactive changes to chemotherapy agents. This finding improves on the second restaging study (the upper panel dated November 6, 2015), providing further evidence of reactive changes.

Teaching Points

1. Focal colonic FDG activity is an abnormal finding commonly seen on oncologic PET-CT scans. Although most of the cases (approximately 90% of them) may represent a benign etiology, primary malignancy or metastasis cannot be ruled out, making further workup warranted. Indeed, this patient underwent biopsy followed by segmental colon resection, both confirming the presence of adenomas without evidence of malignancy.

2. Primary prostate lymphoma (PPL) is an extremely rare extra-nodal NHL confined to the prostate gland. Literatures are scanty with a few case reports only. It appears the main pathological form of PPL is DLBCL, with a favorable response to chemoradiation and a good prognosis. PPL has a high metabolic phenotype different than usually low metabolic phenotype for prostate cancer (adenocarcinoma).

References

Wang C, Jiang P, Ji J. Primary lymphoma of the prostate: two case reports and a review of the literature. Contemp Oncol. 2012;16(5):456–9.

Wang K, Wang N, Sun J, et al. Primary prostate lymphoma: a case report and literature review. Int J Immunopathol Pharmacol. 2019;33 https://doi.org/10.1177/2058738419863217.

Chapter 81
Case 81: PET Superscan

A: Restaging PET-CT in a 74-year-old male with history of prostate carcinoma diagnosed 3 years ago treated with radiation, currently with rising PSA and most recent level of 16.1 ng/mL (normal range of 0.00–2.50). (1) What is the tracer, and where are the normal tracer distribution? (2) What is the PET-CT impression? (3) Is there any evidence of lymphonodal or visceral involvement? If none, what do we recommend in terms of radionuclide-targeted therapy?

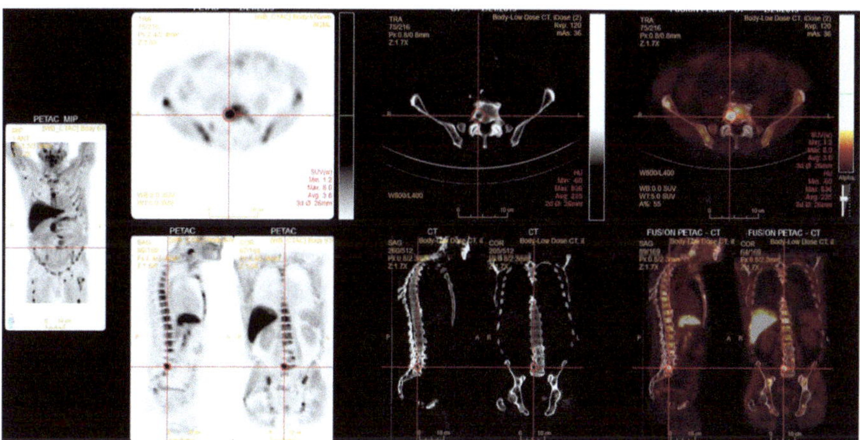

C. Y. O. Wong, D. Wu, *Phenotypic Oncology PET*,
https://doi.org/10.1007/978-3-031-09737-9_81

81.1   Case 81: Interpretation and Teaching

A1:   18F-fluciclovine (Axumin), with normal/physiologic distribution to the liver and the pancreas and often mild/diffuse muscular uptake, with excreted tracer activity in the kidneys and urinary bladder.

A2:   Confluent and asymmetric abnormal tracer uptakes are identified, corresponding to extensive and predominant sclerotic changes mixed with pockets of lytic lesions such as in the right L5 vertebral body (circle of the crosshair), which, in conjunction with rising PSA, is highly suspicious for extensive bony metastatic disease. With the relative lack of tracer activity in the kidneys and urinary bladder, the study is consistent with a superscan due to extensive bony metastases.

A3:   No, there is no definitive evidence for any nodal or visceral involvement. Depending on patient's symptoms, he is a good candidate for Ra-223 (Xofigo) radiation therapy if indicated.

Teaching Point Axumin is a PET radioactive tracer/injection that has been approved by the US FDA for the imaging of suspected prostate cancer recurrence or metastasis based on elevated PSA following treatment. This is an unusual case showing extensive bone metastases with variable Axumin uptake, without normal tracer distribution to the kidneys and urinary bladder, in a pattern consistent with a superscan. The high max SUV of lytic bone lesions indicate a potential rule of Axumin PET-CT in the monitoring of systemic treatment response. According to literature, Axumin PET-CT is superior to whole-body bone scan in both sensitivity and specificity for detection of bone metastases of prostate cancer.

References

Chen B, Wei P, Macapinlac HA, et al. Comparison of 18F-Fluciclovine PET/CT and 99mTc-MDP bone scan in detection of bone metastasis in prostate cancer. Nucl Med Commun. 2019;40(9):940–6.

Li R, Ravizzini GC, Gorin MA, et al. The use of PET CT in prostate cancer. Prostate Cancer Prostate Dis. 2018;21(1):4–21.

Chapter 82
Case 82: Diffuse Idiopathic Pulmonary Neuroendocrine Cell Hyperplasia (DIPNECH)

A: Restaging PET-CT in a 61-year-old female with history of papillary and Hurthle cell thyroid carcinomas status post-completion thyroidectomy 8 months ago followed by radioactive iodide (RAI) therapy with 102.3 mCi of I-131. Diagnostic CT showed multiple bilateral lung nodules, most of them in subcentimeter size, with dominant two nodules, one in the right middle lobe (RML) and another in the left upper lobe (LUL), with recent biopsy-proven RML lung carcinoid tumor and LUL lung neuroendocrine tumor. (1) What is the tracer? (2) What's the normal distribution pattern? (3) What's the PET-CT impression?

C. Y. O. Wong, D. Wu, *Phenotypic Oncology PET*,
https://doi.org/10.1007/978-3-031-09737-9_82

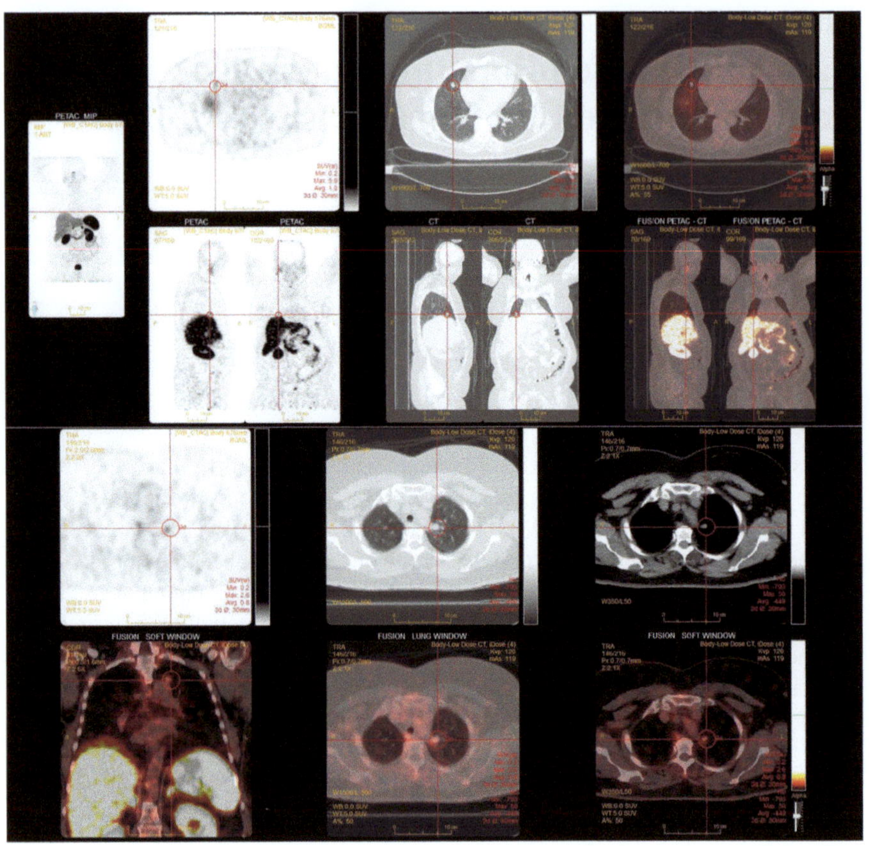

82.1   Case 82: Interpretation and Teaching

A1:   Cu-64 oxodotreotide or DOTATATE.

A2:   Normal distribution of DOTATATE on PET-CT imaging is characterized by mild to moderate uptake by multiple glands including pituitary, salivary, thyroid, and adrenal, but not prostate, and diffuse uptake in the liver and more prominent in the spleen, with excreted tracer activity in the kidneys and urinary bladder.

A3:   The two dominant nodules (RML, about 0.9 cm; LUL, about 0.7 cm) show mild tracer activity, with calculated max SUV of 3.9 and 2.6, respectively, in conjunction with diagnostic CT finding of multiple and bilateral small/tiny pulmonary nodules, consistent with diffuse idiopathic pulmonary neuroendocrine cell hyperplasia (DIPNECH).

Teaching Point Diffuse idiopathic pulmonary neuroendocrine cell hyperplasia (DIPNECH) is a rare lung disease that has a predilection to nonsmoking females in their 60s like this case. Patients with DIPNECH usually present with chronic cough, dyspnea, and CT finding of multiple bilateral small lung nodules with associated mosaic attenuation. DOTATATE PET shall have an additional value in the recognition or detection of DIPNECH due to the DOTATATE avidity in carcinoid or neuroendocrine tumors.

References

Almquist DR, Ernani V, Sonbol MB. Diffuse idiopathic pulmonary neuroendocrine cell hyperplasia: DIPNECH. Curr Opin Pulm Med. 2021;27(4):255–61.

Galffy G. Diagnosis and treatment of the neuroendocrine tumors of the lung. Magy Onkol. 2018;62(2):113–8.

Chapter 83
Case 83: Advanced/Metastatic Ovarian Carcinoma

A: Diagnostic PET-CT in a 45-year-old female with newly developed ascites, status post-paracentesis, and cytology examination pending. Pertinent medical history of left breast cancer (DCIS) treated with lumpectomy, radiation, and maintenance with tamoxifen. New mammogram was unremarkable. CA 15.3 and CA 27.29 were within normal limits; however, CA 125 was elevated to 2853 U/mL with a normal range of 0–21. (1) What is the tracer? (2) Is the ascites FDG positive or negative? (3) What's the PET-CT impression and what do we recommend?

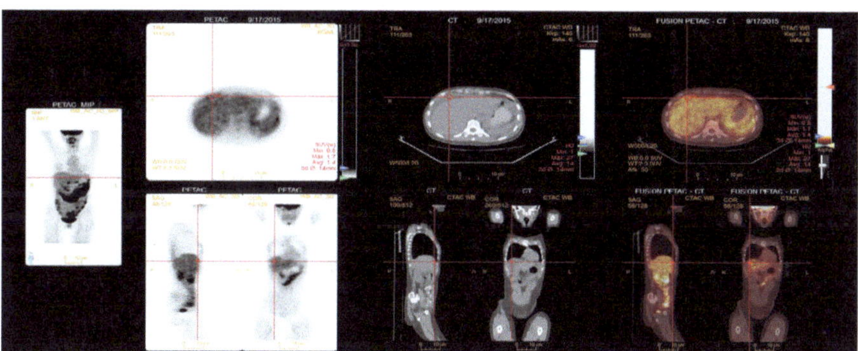

© The Author(s), under exclusive license to Springer Nature Switzerland AG 2022

C. Y. O. Wong, D. Wu, *Phenotypic Oncology PET*, https://doi.org/10.1007/978-3-031-09737-9_83

B: After PET-CT, patient underwent excisional biopsy of the FDG-avid small right axillary node, pathology returned positive for metastatic ovarian carcinoma. She underwent hysterectomy, salpingo-oophorectomy, omentectomy, and total abdominal hysterectomy with staging and debulking, followed by systemic and intra-abdominal chemotherapy. Repeated laboratory tests show CA 125 dropped to lowest 25 U/mL from the peak level of 7793. However, CA 125 gradually rose despite multiple rounds of clinical trials and conventional chemotherapy. Diagnostic CTs showed persistent para-rectal mass. Restaging PET-CTs were performed. (1) What is new on PET images? (2) What are PET-CT impression and prognosis?

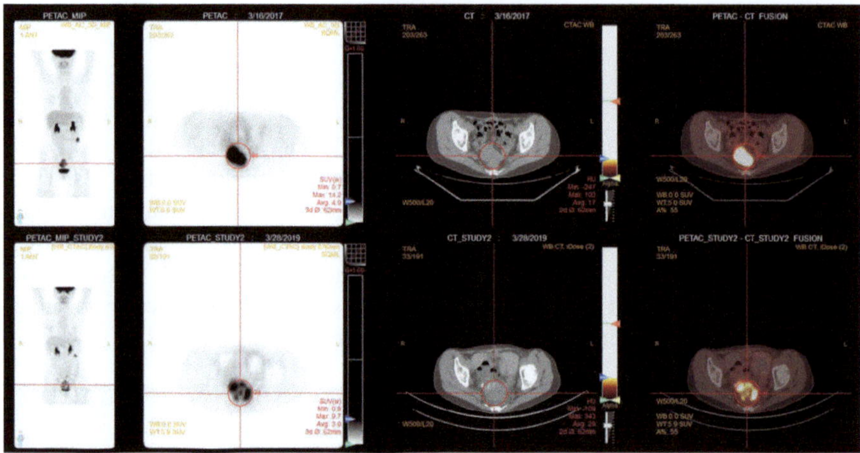

83.1   Case 83: Interpretation and Teaching

A1:   F-18 FDG.

A2:   Yes, there is mild FDG activity corresponding to ascites in right upper abdomen, max SUV at 1.7, suspicious for malignant ascites.

A3:   There is an irregular FDG-avid pelvis mass. Diffuse FDG activity is noted likely corresponding the omentum, concerning for early stage of abdominal carcinomatosis. Also, there is focal and mild FDG activity, corresponding to a small node in the right axillary region and the right internal mammary region, suspicious for nodal metastasis. Further workup including biopsy for definitive diagnosis shall be recommended.

B1:   In addition to an FDG-avid para-rectal/presacral mass, there is an FDG-avid peri-colonic mass in the left abdomen; both are highly suspicious for metastases.

B2:   Despite continued clinical trials and conventional chemotherapy, the persistent two metastatic masses show a poor response, indicating chemoresistant metastatic ovarian cancer, with a poor prognosis.

Teaching Point   Ovarian carcinoma remains the leading cause of death from gynecological malignancies. Most of the cases are diagnosed at advanced stage like in this case. Although initial treatment response is often very good, approximately 90–95% of patients with stage IV ovarian cancer experience relapse despite continued treatments, as shown in this patient. All the patients with newly diagnosed ovarian cancer shall have genetic consultation and test. This patient was found to have BRCA1 germline mutation, which helped in the selection of clinical trial/maintenance therapy with Olaparib, inhibiting poly(ADP-ribose) polymerase (PARP), an enzyme involved in DNA repair, although the response/prognosis might still be poor.

References

Antunovic L, Cimitan M, Borsatti E, et al. Revisiting the clinical value of 18F-FDG PET/CT in detection of recurrent epithelial ovarian carcinomas: correlation with histology, serum CA-125 assay, and conventional radiological modalities. Clin Nucl Med. 2012;37(8):e184–8.

Khiewvan B, Torigian DA, Emamzadehfard S, et al. An update on the role of PET/CT and PET/MRI in ovarian cancer. Eur J Nucl Med Mol Imaging. 2017;44(6):1079–91.

Chapter 84
Case 84: Metastatic Prostate Cancer or Neuroendocrine Tumor?

A: Restaging PET-CT in a 66-year-old male with history of prostate cancer, treated with prostatectomy and radiation 9 years ago, currently with slightly elevated PSA, at a level of 0.78 ng/mL from prior 0.65 ng/mL half a year ago. (1) What is the tracer? (2) What do we recommend?

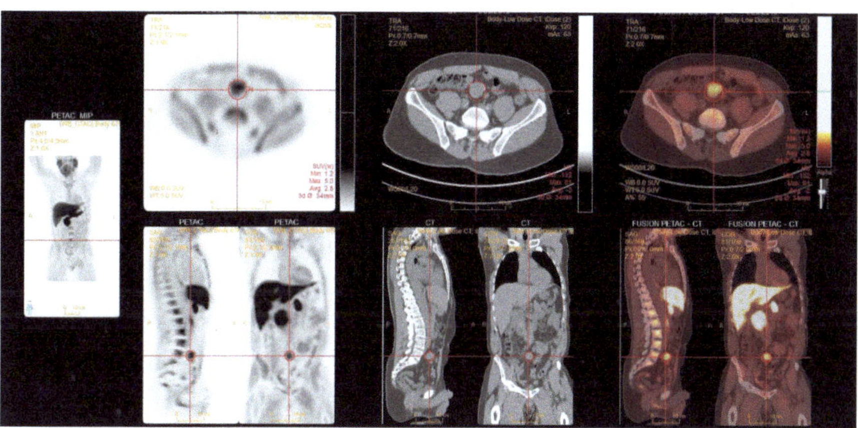

C. Y. O. Wong, D. Wu, *Phenotypic Oncology PET*,
https://doi.org/10.1007/978-3-031-09737-9_84

B: Patient underwent a CT-guided biopsy of the pelvic mass with pathology returned positive for low-grade neuroendocrine tumor. Subsequently, a new PET-CT was performed. (1) What is the tracer? (2) Is there any evidence for primary neuroendocrine tumor? (3) Is there any evidence for lesions additional to the known central pelvic mass?

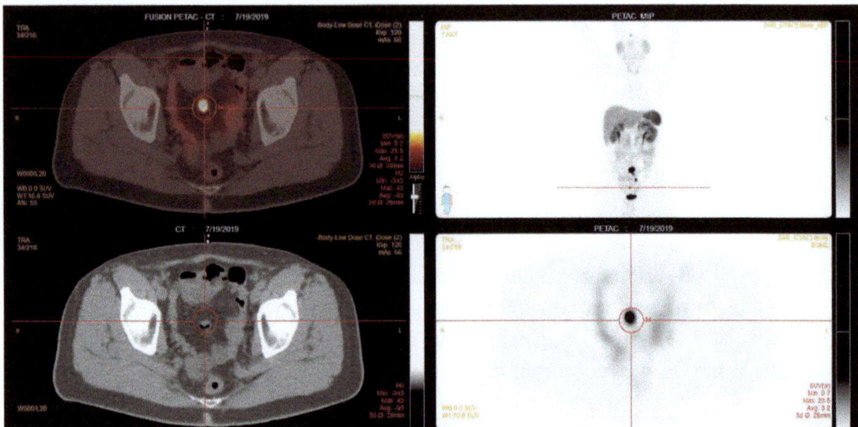

84.1 Case 84: Interpretation and Teaching

A1: Axumin (18F-fluciclovine).

A2: There is an approximately 3.2 × 2.9 cm soft tissue mass in the central pelvis with moderate Axumin uptake, suspicious for metastatic prostate cancer. Recommend biopsy for definitive diagnosis.

B1: Ga-68 DOTATATE.

B2: Yes, there is focal DOTATATE uptake correlated to focal thickened small intestine wall in the anterior aspect (circle of the crosshair), suspicious for ileum primary neuroendocrine tumor.

B3: Images confirm the central pelvic mass with intense DOTATATE uptake, consistent with biopsy-proven neuroendocrine tumor. In addition, there are at least two small foci, one in the left pelvis and another superior anterior to the urine bladder, both suspicious for neuroendocrine tumor. Two months after the positive Ga-68 DOTATATE PET-CT study, patient underwent small intestine (distal ileum) segmental resection confirming intestinal neuroendocrine tumor and mesenteric lymph node dissection confirming four out of eight positive for neuroendocrine tumor.

Teaching Point Axumin (18F-fluciclovine) is an FDA-approved radioactive tracer for PET imaging of patients with suspected metastatic or recurrent prostate cancer. So far, there are only a couple of case reports about Axumin uptake by neuroendocrine tumor. Further molecular imaging with Ga-68 DOTATATE PET CT not only confirms the biopsy-proven central pelvic neuroendocrine mass but also demonstrates focal activity in small intestine suggesting primary and additional small nodal lesions in the adjacent pelvic regions, leading to successful surgical resection of the small intestinal primary tumor and multiple mesenteric metastases.

References

Abiodun-Ojo OA, Akintayo AA, Harik LR, et al. Poorly differentiated neuroendocrine tumor with 18F-fluciclovine uptake in a patient with metastatic castrate-resistant prostate cancer. Clin Nucl Med. 2021;46(5):e282–5.

Balazova Z, Cerny I, Vyskvsky P. Incidental accumulation of fluciclovine in neuroendocrine tumor in a patient with oncological duplicity. Case rep Oncologia. 2020;13(1):431–5.

Chapter 85
Case 85: Metastatic Thyroid Carcinoma

A: Restaging PET-CT with Thyrogen stimulation in an 83-year-old male with history of papillary thyroid carcinoma, treated with total thyroidectomy and RAI 10 years ago, now with rising thyroglobulin levels. Laboratory test showed TSH 137.82 following two Thyrogen injections, stimulated thyroglobulin 245.0, and thyroglobulin antibody <20. (1) What is the tracer? (2) What is the PET-CT impression?

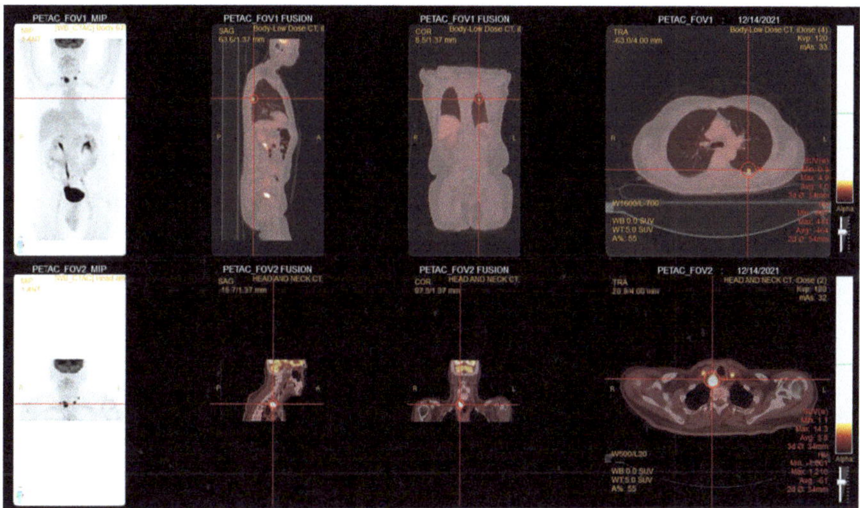

C. Y. O. Wong, D. Wu, *Phenotypic Oncology PET*, https://doi.org/10.1007/978-3-031-09737-9_85

B: Patient also underwent I-131 neck/chest whole-body scan, with SPECT-CT images as the following: (1) Is there any I-131 avid lesion in the neck? (2) Is the left lung nodule I-131 avid? (3) What's the implication in RAI decision-making?

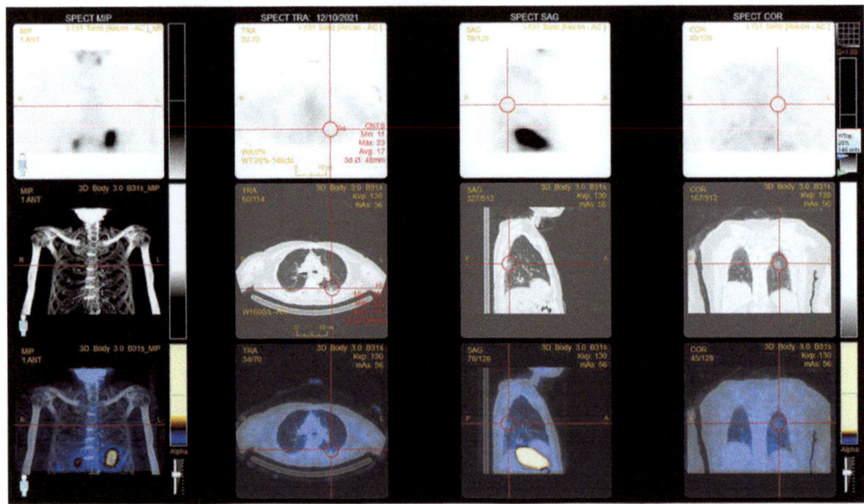

85.1 Case 85: Interpretation and Teaching

A1: F-18 FDG.

A2: FDG PET-CT identifies four foci with variable activities involving bilateral lower/inferior neck and one FDG-avid left lower lobe (LLL) lung nodule, in conjunction with the markedly elevated thyroglobulin under Thyrogen stimulation, highly suspicious for locoregional lymphonodal and left lung metastases of thyroid origin.

B1: No, the whole-body images (data not shown) and dedicated neck/chest images with SPECT-CT show no discrete appreciable I-131 accumulation to correspond to the four FDG-avid lesions in the neck region.

B2: No, the SPECT-CT images redemonstrate a subcentimeter pulmonary nodule in the posterior aspect of the LLL (circle of the crosshair), without appreciable I-131 uptake.

B3: The discordant findings between FDG PET-CT and I-131 scan, with positive FDG lesions but negative I-131 avidity, are typical for de-differentiated metastatic/recurrent thyroid carcinomas, indicating a limited role of RAI for therapy. Therefore, other treatment options, such as surgical resection, chemotherapy, or radiation, should be explored, mainly depending on new biopsy results, other coexisting conditions, and patient's and treating physician's preference.

Teaching Point FDG PET-CT has been increasingly utilized for restaging of metastatic/recurrent thyroid carcinomas. This is optimally performed with thyroid withdrawal or Thyrogen stimulation as shown in this case, with an overall improved sensitivity. The discordant findings of FDG-avid lesions but without I-131 accumulation effectively exclude RAI as an option of future treatment. Biopsy of representative lesions is routinely recommended, due to clinical concerns of anaplastic or poorly differentiated thyroid cancers, although markedly elevated thyroglobulin is suggestive of de-differentiated thyroid carcinoma. Cases of this kind shall be presented and discussed for multidisciplinary consideration for best approach and optimal therapies.

References

Manohar PM, Beesley LJ, Bellile EL, et al. Prognostic value of FDG PET/CT metabolic parameters in metastatic radioiodine-refractory differentiated thyroid cancer. Clin Nucl Med. 2018;43(9):641–7.

Zampella E, Klain M, Pace L, et al. PET/CT in the management of differentiated thyroid cancer. Diagn Interv Imaging. 2021;102(9):515–23.

Chapter 86
Case 86: Primary Breast Carcinoma or Metastatic Neuroendocrine Carcinoma to the Breast?

A: PET-CT in a 71-year-old female with biopsy-proven invasive ductal carcinoma of both breasts. (1) What is the tracer? (2) Is the PET finding typical for invasive ductal breast carcinoma? (3) What do we recommend regarding the FDG-avid left upper lobe (LUL)/supra-hilar lesion?

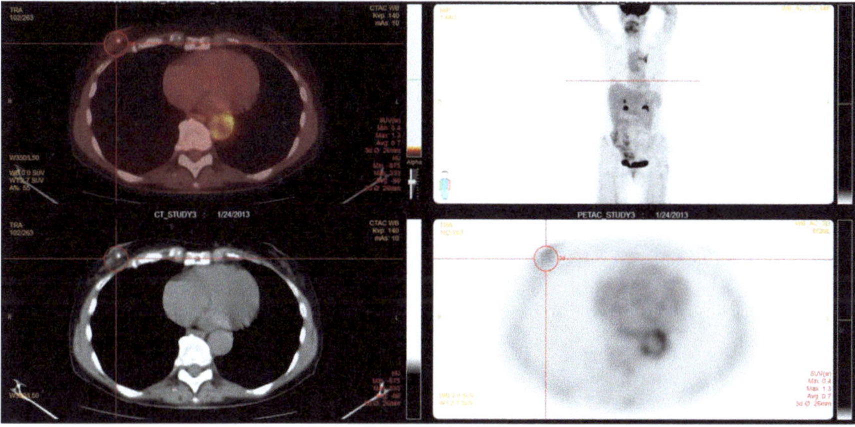

© The Author(s), under exclusive license to Springer Nature
Switzerland AG 2022
C. Y. O. Wong, D. Wu, *Phenotypic Oncology PET*,
https://doi.org/10.1007/978-3-031-09737-9_86

B: Further expert review of the breast biopsies specimen indicates carcinoma with neuroendocrine features. Core biopsy of the FDG-avid LUL lung nodule returned positive for neuroendocrine carcinoma (atypical carcinoid tumor). Restaging PET-CT was performed after completion of chemo radiation. (1) What's the response to chemo radiation?

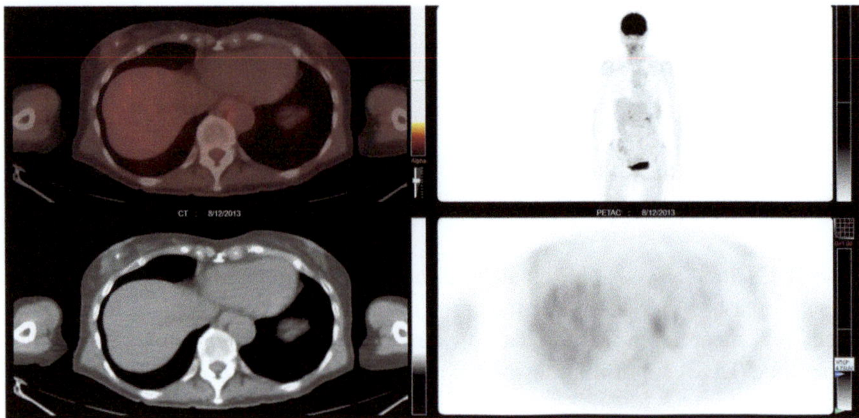

86.1 Case 86: Interpretation and Teaching

A1: F-18 FDG.
A2: No. Invasive ductal breast carcinomas often show moderate FDG activity on PET-CT imaging, relative to mild activity in typical lobular breast carcinomas or carcinoid/neuroendocrine tumors. In this case, there are at least two right breast lesions, both with mild FDG activity, max SUV only 1.3. Although biopsy was reported to be left breast invasive ductal carcinoma, there is no appreciable discrete FDG activity in the left breast region. In contrast, there is a LLL lung nodule with higher FDG activity, max SUV 4.8, suspicious for lung primary malignancy. Also, there is an FDG-avid right liver lesion (data not shown), concerning for intrahepatic metastasis.
A3: Biopsy of the LLL lung lesion for definite diagnosis shall be recommended.
B1: The response to chemo radiation is excellent, with decreased metabolic activity in all lesions, including the LLL lung primary, the two right breast lesions, and the known right liver lesion (data not shown). Of note, whole brain was included on the restaging PET-CT, due to MRI brain showing findings suspicious for multiple micro-hemorrhagic metastases. There is no discrete abnormal FDG activity in the brain suggestive of metastasis, however, due to small size or low uptake relative to neuronal uptake.

Teaching Point Metastatic neuroendocrine carcinomas could involve multiple organs or tissues, often characterized by minimal to mild FDG activity on PET-CT imaging. Morphological and pathologically, metastatic neuroendocrine tumors to the breast can mimic primary mammary breast carcinomas. Any atypical features on FDG PET-CT for primary breast carcinomas despite pathological diagnosis as shown in this case shall raise concerns for further investigation, including biopsy of more metabolically active lesion(s) for definite diagnosis.

References

Economopoulou P. Breast metastasis from neuroendocrine carcinoma of the lung. Case Rep Oncol. 2020;13:1281–4.

Perry KD, Reynolds C, Rose DG, et al. Metastatic neuroendocrine tumour in the breast: a potential mimic of in-situ and invasive mammary carcinoma. Histopathol. 2011;59(4):619–30.

Chapter 87
Case 87: Atypical Oligometastasis of Malignant Melanoma

A: Restaging PET-CT in a 62-year-old female with newly diagnosed malignant melanoma of lateral left thigh status post-excision 2 weeks ago. (1) What is the tracer? (2) What is the impression about the excision site? (3) Is there any evidence of metastasis?

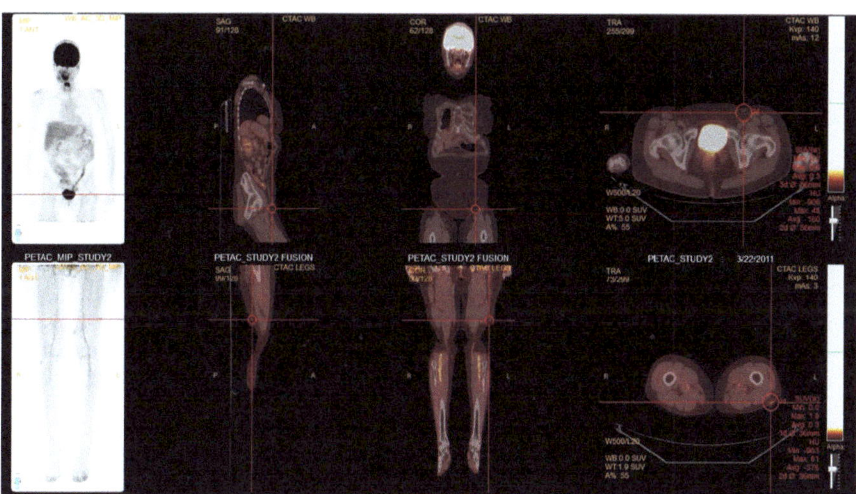

C. Y. O. Wong, D. Wu, *Phenotypic Oncology PET*,
https://doi.org/10.1007/978-3-031-09737-9_87

B: Patient did not have any chemo radiation or immunotherapy. Surveillance PET-CT scans were performed. (1) Is there any evidence of recurrence at the left thigh primary site? (2) What do we recommend regarding the left deep upper back lesion?

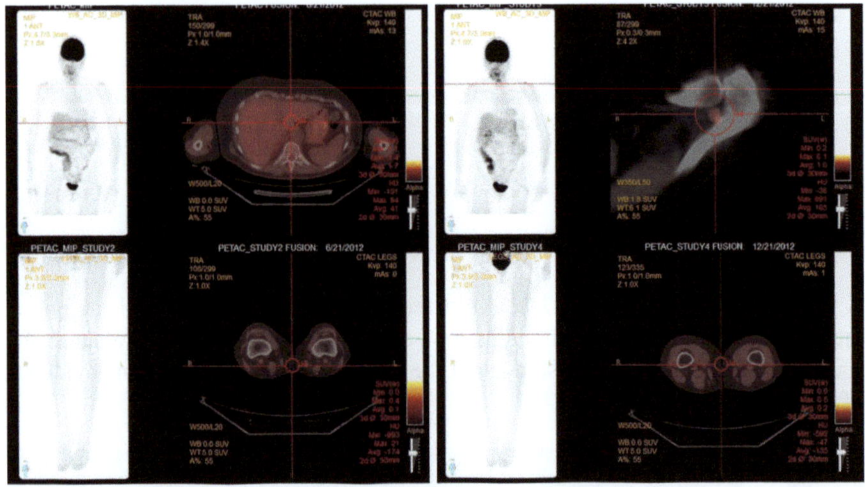

87.1   Case 87: Interpretation and Teaching

A1:   F-18 FDG.
A2:   There is minimal FDG activity on the surface of the excision site, without CT correlate for nodularity or mass, in favor of postsurgical/inflammatory changes.
A3:   There is no discrete abnormal FDG activity in the remainder of the whole-body PET scan to suggest metastasis.
B1:   Surveillance PET-CT scans showed no evidence of FDG-avid residual or recurrent disease at the left thigh primary site.
B2:   The second surveillance PET-CT (the right pane), however, shows an approximately 0.5 cm round-shaped soft tissue lesion with moderate FDG activity, max SUV 6.1, located deeply between the left clavicular bone and lateral left scapular in the upper left back, suspicious for atypical metastasis, for which biopsy shall be recommended for definite diagnosis. Indeed, the patient underwent a biopsy of the left upper back lesion 1 month later, with pathology returned positive for metastatic melanoma.

Teaching Point This is a unique case showing atypical but biopsy-proven oligo-metastasis of malignant melanoma. Given the deep location between the left clavicular bone and scapula, it's atypical for a site of lymphonodal metastasis but instead suggestive of hematogenic dissemination or seeding, which is often associated with a grim prognosis. This has been confirmed by subsequently developed metastases to the lung and brain, despite multiple cycles of immunotherapy with Yervoy (ipilimumab) and gamma knife treatments.

References

Bisschop C, de Heer EC, Brouwers AH, et al. Rational use of 18F-FDG PET CT in patients with advanced cutaneous melanoma: a systematic review. Crit Rev. Oncol Hematol. 2020;153:103044.

Fares J, Fares MY, Khachfe HH, et al. Molecular principles of metastasis: a hallmark of cancer revisited. Signal Transduct Target Ther. 2020;5:28.

Chapter 88
Case 88: Dual-Time PET-CT Evaluation of Lung Nodules

A: Diagnostic PET-CT in a 59-year-old female with extensive history of smoking, and serial CTs showing interval enlarged right lower lobe (RLL) lung nodule (current 0.84×0.54 cm versus prior 0.65×0.40 cm). A dual-time imaging protocol was utilized, with a 75-minute apart between the initial eye-to-thigh PET-CT and delayed/dedicated chest PET CT. Patient's blood glucose level was 73 mg/dL. (1) What is the tracer? (2) What's PET-CT impression about the RLL nodule? (3) Is there any evidence of metastasis to the hila or mediastinum? (4) What's likely cause of the right colonic tracer uptake, and why?

© The Author(s), under exclusive license to Springer Nature
Switzerland AG 2022
C. Y. O. Wong, D. Wu, *Phenotypic Oncology PET*,
https://doi.org/10.1007/978-3-031-09737-9_88

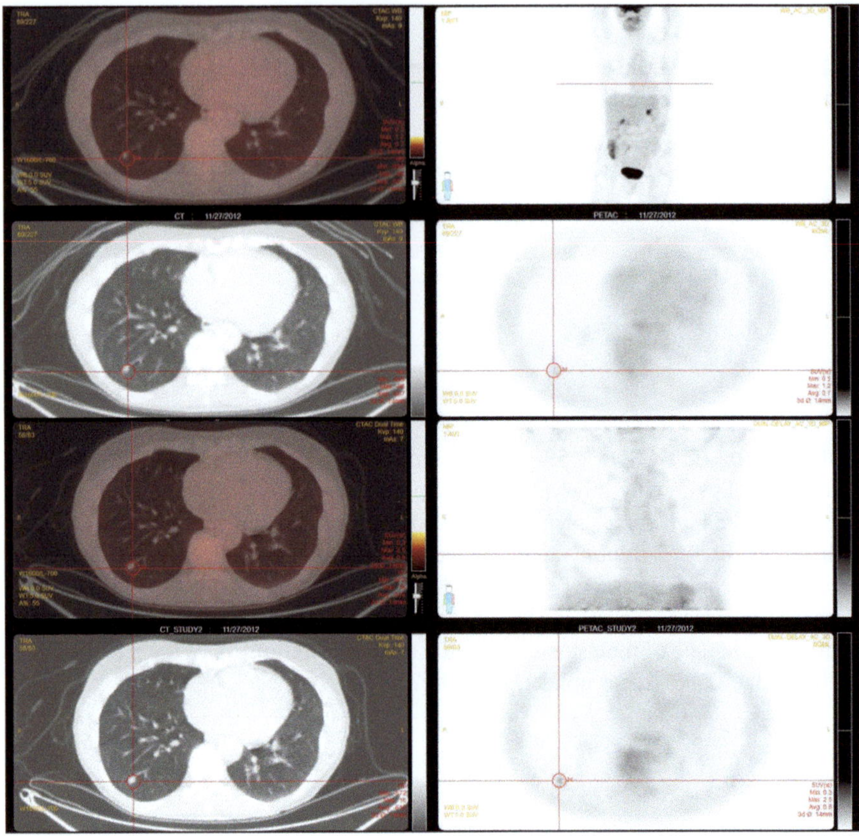

88.1   Case 88: Interpretation and Teaching

A1:   F-18 FDG.

A2:   Despite the subcentimeter size, the RLL nodule of concern shows mild FDG activity on initial regular PET imaging, which increases on the delayed imaging, calculated max SUV 1.2 on initial and 2.5 on delayed imaging, respectively, indicating a 108% increment in metabolic activity. The PET feature, in conjunction with CT evidence of interval growth and extensive smoking history, is suspicious for right lung primary malignancy with a low metabolic rate.

A3:   There is no discrete abnormal FDG activity or CT finding to suggest metastasis to the hila or mediastinum.

A4:   There is vertical linear/elongated FDG activity noted in the proximal ascending colon/cecum, in a diffuse pattern suggestive of a physiologic or benign etiology. The ascending colon often has more prominent FDG activity relative to the other parts of the colorectal tract in general.

Teaching Point Dual-time FDG PET-CT had been introduced about two decades ago to improve evaluation of pulmonary nodules. This imaging protocol has not been widely accepted or adopted, due to a variety of reasons. This case demonstrates a unique value of dual-time FDG PET-CT in selected patients and significantly increases reading physician's confidence to call a positive study, for which biopsy for definite diagnosis is recommended instead of further imaging follow-up. Two months later, the patient underwent RLL lobectomy and lymph node dissection. Pathology exam confirmed a 0.9 cm poor-differentiated adenocarcinoma, corresponding to the FDG-avid nodule with 108% increased metabolic activity on delayed PET imaging. Also, there is a 0.3 cm RLL nodule that is apparently non-FDG-avid, but positive for moderately differentiated adenocarcinoma. Eight nodes were collected, all negative for metastasis. In summary, the appropriate impression of FDG PET-CT shall be suspicious for RLL lung primary malignancy with a low metabolic rate.

References

Alkhawaldeh K, Bural G, Kumar R, Alavi A. Impact of dual-time-point (18)F-FDG PET imaging and partial volume correction in the assessment of solitary pulmonary nodules. Eur J Nucl Med Mol Imaging. 2008;35(2):246–52.

Zhang L, Wang Y, Lei J, et al. Dual time point 18F-FDG PET/CT versus single time point 18F-FDG PET/CT for the differential diagnosis of pulmonary nodules: a meta-analysis. Acta Radiol. 2013;54(7):770–7.

Chapter 89
Case 89: Combined Phenotypes
of Pulmonary Large-Cell Neuroendocrine
Carcinoma (LCNEC) and Squamous Cell
Carcinoma (SCC)

A: Initial staging PET-CT in a 62-year-old female with newly diagnosed neuroendocrine carcinoma (atypical carcinoid tumor) of the right lung. (1) What is the tracer? (2) Is the right lower lobe (RLL) lesion's tracer intensity typical for neuroendocrine tumors? (3) Is there any evidence of metastasis to the hila or mediastinum?

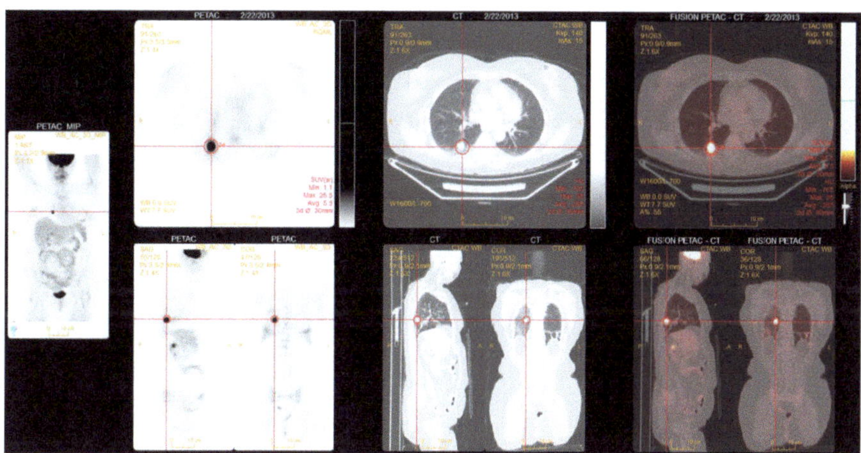

C. Y. O. Wong, D. Wu, *Phenotypic Oncology PET*,
https://doi.org/10.1007/978-3-031-09737-9_89

89.1   Case 89: Interpretation and Teaching

A1:   F-18 FDG.

A2:   No. Neuroendocrine carcinoma (NEC) or carcinoid tumors typically exhibit mild to moderate FDG activity on PET-CT imaging. The solidary pulmonary nodule of the RLL shows intensive FDG uptake, max SUV 25.5, inconsistent with the pathological diagnosis. Further workup shall be recommended.

A3:   No, there is no discrete abnormal FDG activity to suggest metastasis to hila or mediastinum.

Teaching Point   This case demonstrates discrepancy between diagnostic pathology and FDG PET metabolic tumor phenotypic patterns. It's well known that primary NECs often exhibit mild to moderate FDG activity on PET imaging. Intense uptake with max SUV of 25.5 is atypical and requires further workup if warranted. This patient underwent mediastinoscopy and lymph node biopsies, all negative for metastasis. Subsequently, she underwent RLL lobectomy and hilar/interlobar lymph node dissection. Pathology returned positive for combined high-grade large cell neuroendocrine carcinoma (LCNEC) and squamous cell carcinoma (SCC), all the 11 nodes negative for metastasis. Patient completed chemotherapy; clinical observation and CT imaging surveillance have shown no evidence of recurrent or metastatic disease over the last 9 years.

References

Oda R, Okuda K, Yamashita Y, et al. Long-term survivor of pulmonary combined large cell neuroendocrine carcinoma treated with nivolumab. Thorac Cancer. 2020;11(7):2036–9.

Rossi G, Bisagni A, Cavazza A. High-grade neuroendocrine carcinoma. Curr Opin Pulm Med. 2014;20(4):332–9.

Yamada K, Maeshima AM, Tsuta K, et al. Combined high-grade neuroendocrine carcinoma of the lung: clinicopathological and immunohistochemical study of 34 surgically resected cases. Pathol Intl. 2014;64(1):28–33.

Chapter 90
Case 90: Primary Nodular Pulmonary Amyloidosis

A: Diagnostic dual-time PET-CT in an 82-year-old male with CT finding of multiple bilateral lung nodules. Pertinent medical history of pulmonary amyloidosis and rheumatoid arthritis. (1) What is the tracer? (2) What's PET-CT impression?

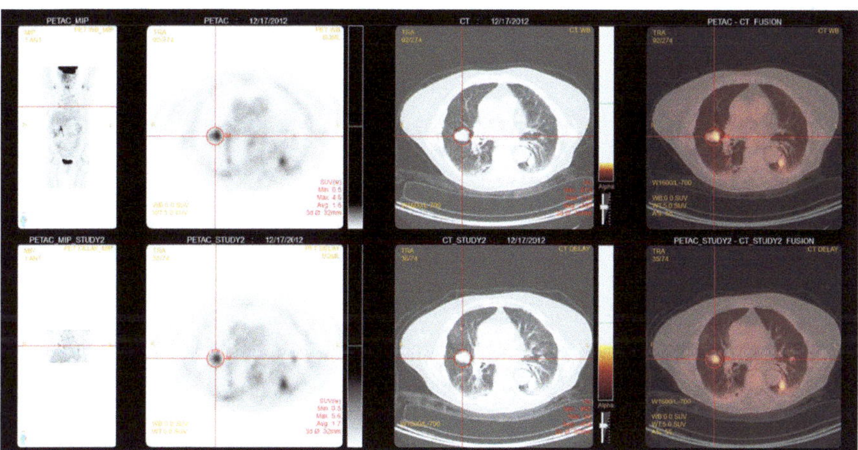

© The Author(s), under exclusive license to Springer Nature Switzerland AG 2022

C. Y. O. Wong, D. Wu, *Phenotypic Oncology PET*,

https://doi.org/10.1007/978-3-031-09737-9_90

B: Half a year later, another diagnostic PET-CT was performed with images displayed in the lower panel in comparison to the aforementioned PET-CT images (upper panel). (1) Is there tracer intensity change on the follow-up PET-CT scan? (2) How was the overall pattern suggesting the diagnosis?

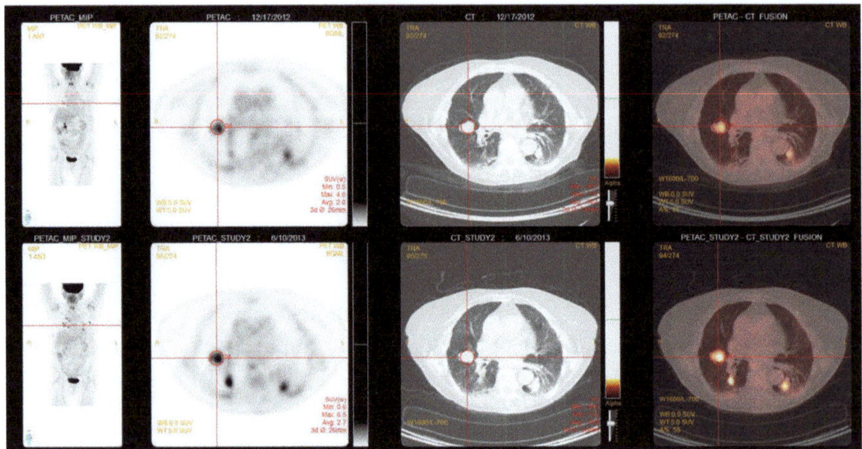

90.1 Case 90: Interpretation and Teaching

A1:   F-18 FDG.

A2:   Redemonstrated are multiple pulmonary nodules involving both lungs, with abnormal FDG activity that was further increased on the delayed PET imaging, mimicking malignancy, or metastasis. However, given the known history of amyloidosis, the overall findings are still consistent with nodular amyloidosis with variable metabolic activities, although coexisting or underlying malignancy cannot be excluded. Further workup including biopsy for definite diagnosis is recommended if clinically warranted.

B1:   Yes, in comparison to the first PET-CT (dated December 17, 2012, the upper panel), near all the nodules on the follow-up study (dated June 10, 2013, the lower panel) show persistently increased FDG activity.

B2:   However, the overall pattern is stable. The sizes of the bilateral lung nodules are essentially stable, despite across-board increased metabolic activity. Therefore, the imaging impression is still nodular pulmonary amyloidosis with possible flaring inflammatory changes.

Teaching Point Amyloidosis is a rare condition caused by a buildup of abnormal amyloid deposits in many organs or parts of the human body. Primary pulmonary amyloidosis comprises three different clinicopathologic types: diffuse alveolar-septal amyloidosis, nodular pulmonary amyloidosis, and tracheobronchial amyloidosis. Among them, primary nodular pulmonary amyloidosis often poses challenge in clinical diagnostic PET-CT evaluation. As shown in this case, increased FDG activity can occur on the delayed PET imaging, limiting the value of dual-time PET-CT imaging protocol. On follow-up PET-CT studies, flaring inflammation of the amyloid nodules can exhibit increased or fluctuating metabolic activity, mimicking malignancy, or metastasis. Careful history review and correlation with prior chest radiographic studies shall be very helpful.

In addition to PET, classic nodular pulmonary amyloidosis often has all or part of the following CT features: very sharp or lobulated nodules; macro- or microcalcifications; varying sizes from 0.5 to 15.0 cm; very slow growth; and surrounding bronchovascular structures.

References

Baqir M, Lowe V, Yi ES, Ryu JH. 18F-FDG PET scanning in pulmonary amyloidosis. J Nucl Med. 2014;55(4):565–8.

Dong MJ, Zhao K, Liu ZF, et al. Primary pulmonary amyloidosis misdiagnosed as malignancy on dual-time-point fluoro-deoxyglucose positron emission tomography/computed tomography: a case report and review of literature. Oncol Lett. 2015;9(2):591–4.

Chapter 91
Case 91: Advanced Follicular Dendritic Cell Sarcoma (FDCS)

A: Initial staging PET-CT in a 73-year-old male with newly diagnosed follicular dendritic cell sarcoma (FDCS) via excisional biopsy of left axillary node. (1) What is the tracer? (2) Are there any technical limitations in the PET-CT study? (3) Is the pleural effusion positive or negative on PET?

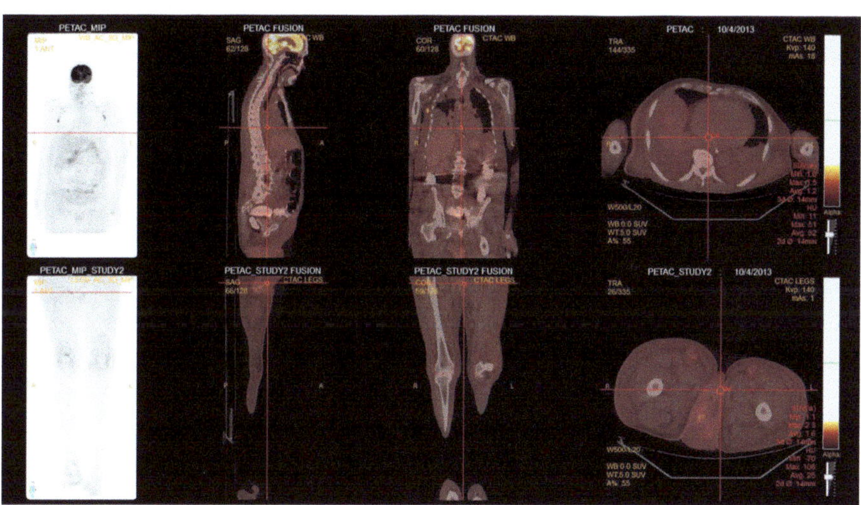

C. Y. O. Wong, D. Wu, *Phenotypic Oncology PET*,
https://doi.org/10.1007/978-3-031-09737-9_91

B: Due to multiple comorbidities, patient received six cycles of reduced dose CHOP (25% less) in 5 months. Restaging PET-CT scans were performed for monitoring treatment response and for surveillance. (1) What is the response to reduced dose CHOP chemotherapy? (2) What is the impression of the last PET-CT (far-right panel)? (3) Is there any splenic involvement? (4) What is the likely cause of right wrist/hand FDG activity?

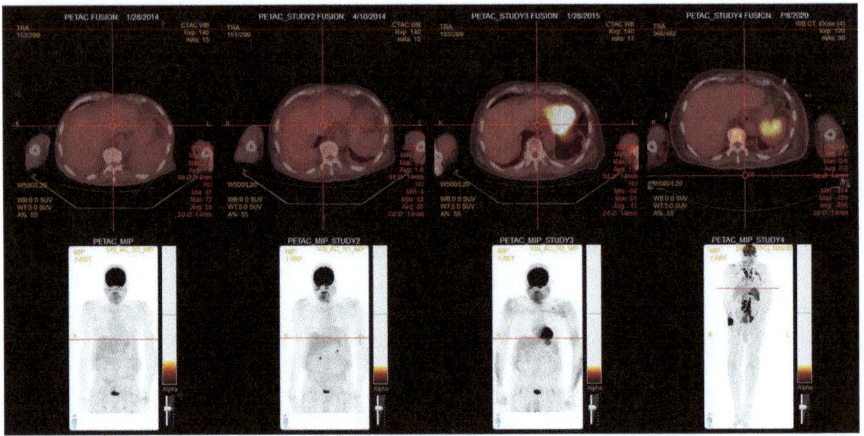

91.1   Case 91: Interpretation and Teaching

A1:   F-18 FDG.

A2:   Yes. The PET-CT is technically limited due to diffuse soft tissue tracer uptake likely secondary to anasarca, bilateral pleural effusions, and ascites. Therefore, the measured max SUVs are likely underestimated.

A3:   No, there is no appreciable FDG activity in bilateral pleural effusions or ascites (data not shown), in favor of benign effusions/ascites, which was confirmed by negative paracentesis and cytology examination. Half a year later, bone marrow biopsy was also negative for involvement.

B1:   The response to reduced dose CHOP was excellent, with steady improvement of not only the adenopathy above and below the diaphragm but also the pleural effusions and ascites.

B2:   However, the last PET-CT (far-right panel) dated August 8, 2020, shows extensive FDG adenopathy above and below the diaphragm, highly suggestive of recurrent disease, which was biopsied, via an excisional biopsy of left axillary lymph node, confirming the diagnosis.

B3:   Yes, in addition to extensive lymphonodal involvement, there is abnormal and heterogeneous FDG activity in the normal-sized spleen, suspicious for extra nodal splenic involvement.

B4:   The diffuse FDG activity in the right wrist/hand region is most likely due to tracer infiltration from injection site.

Teaching Point Follicular dendritic cell sarcoma (FDCS) is a rare malignancy often arising from lymph nodes, later involving extra nodal tissue or organ, as shown in this case. FDCS is an aggressive malignant tumor, with a poor prognosis. Patients with FDCS may have a good response to standard chemotherapy with CHOP; however, many of them (more than 81%) relapse in a few years. Therefore, the clinical course of this case is typical, in line with literature.

References

Wu A, Pullarkat S. Follicular dendritic cell sarcoma. Arch Pathol Lab Med. 2016;140(2):186–90.

Youens KE, Waugh MS. Extranodal follicular dendritic cell sarcoma. Arch Pathol Lab Med. 2008;132(10):1683–7.

Chapter 92
Case 92: Oligometastatic Prostate Cancer

A: Restaging PET-CT in a 68-year-old male patient with history of Gleason 8 prostate carcinoma, treated with radical robotic prostatectomy, salvage radiation, hormone therapy (Lupron injections), and currently on oral chemotherapy. Most recent PSA level was 0.7 ng/mL on February 2, 2019, rising from the prior PSA of <0.1 ng/mL on September 26, 2018. (1) What is the tracer? (2) What sign does the PET imaging resemble in the head and neck region? (3) What's the likely cause of the mild tracer uptake in the center of bilateral breasts? (4) There are three small foci and one moderate-sized focus of tracer in the lateral of the right abdomen wall and right thigh. What's the likely cause of the findings? (5) What is the PET-CT impression about the right posterior iliac lesion? (6) Is there any evidence of additional metastatic or malignant involvement?

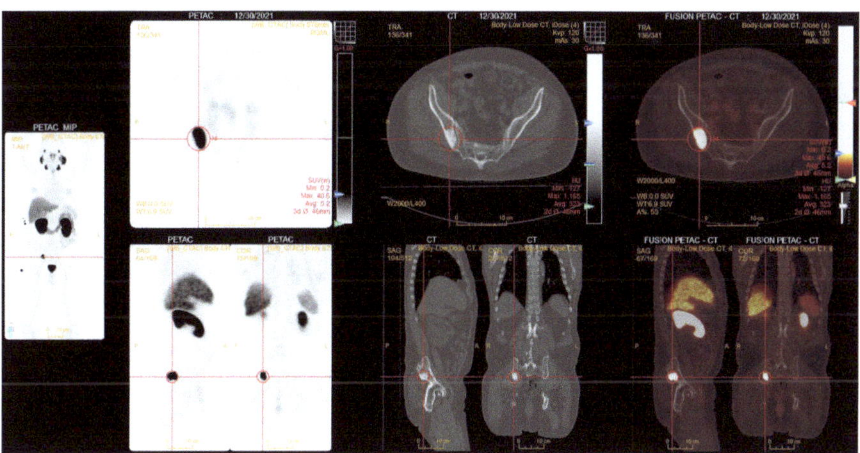

C. Y. O. Wong, D. Wu, *Phenotypic Oncology PET*,
https://doi.org/10.1007/978-3-031-09737-9_92

92.1   Case 92: Interpretation and Teaching

A1:   F18-PSMA (PYLARIFY).

A2:   Due to normal tracer distribution to the bilateral lacrimal glands, the nasal cavity, the bilateral parotid, and submandibular salivary glands, the findings in the head/neck resemble a "panda sign."

A3:   The mild tracer uptake in bilateral nipples is likely due to gynecomastia.

A4:   The three foci in a linear pattern and a single focus in the lateral of the abdomen wall and thigh are most likely due to tracer contamination.

A5:   There is an approximately 3.2 × 2.0 cm sclerotic lesion in the posterior right iliac bone, with intense tracer uptake, max SUV 40.6, suspicious for a site of bony metastasis from the prostate carcinoma.

A6:   No, there is normal tracer distribution to the liver and spleen, with excreted tracer activity in the kidneys and the urinary bladder.

Teaching Point F18-PSMA (PYLarify) is the second generation of prostate-specific membrane antigen (PSMA)-based positron emission tracer that FDA approved for PET imaging of suspected metastasis or recurrence of prostate cancer. Demonstrated in this case is a single bone lesion with sclerotic changes on CT, but intense tracer uptake is seen with max SUV 40.6. The significance of high PSMA avidity of sclerotic bone metastasis is of at least twofold: 1. F18-PSMA PET-CT probably not only has higher specificity but also higher sensitivity in the detection of metastatic or recurrent bone metastasis of prostate cancer, in comparison to conventional CT, bone scan, or FDG PET-CT. 2. The intense tracer activity of bone metastasis could be utilized as a baseline for monitoring treatment response.

References

Pianou NK, Stavrou PZ, Vlontzou E, et al. More advantages in detecting bone and soft tissue metastases from prostate cancer using (18)F-PSMA PET CT. Hell J Nucl Med. 2019;22(1):6–9.

Rowe SP, Macura KJ, Mena E, et al. PSMA-based [18F]DCFPyL PET CT is superior to conventional imaging for lesion detection in patients with metastatic prostate cancer. Mol Imaging Biol. 2016;18(3):411–9.

Chapter 93
Case 93: Bulky Primary Mediastinal Lymphoma

A: Diagnostic PET-CT in a 58-year-old female patient presented with superior vena cava (SVC) syndrome, apparently caused by a large mediastinal mass (15 × 11 × 14 cm), status post-CT-guided biopsy with pathology pending. (1) What is the tracer? (2) Does the mediastinal lesion meet criteria of bulky disease? (3) Is there any lesion other than the mediastinal mass? (4) Max SUV of the left pleural effusion is 0.8; what do we recommend?

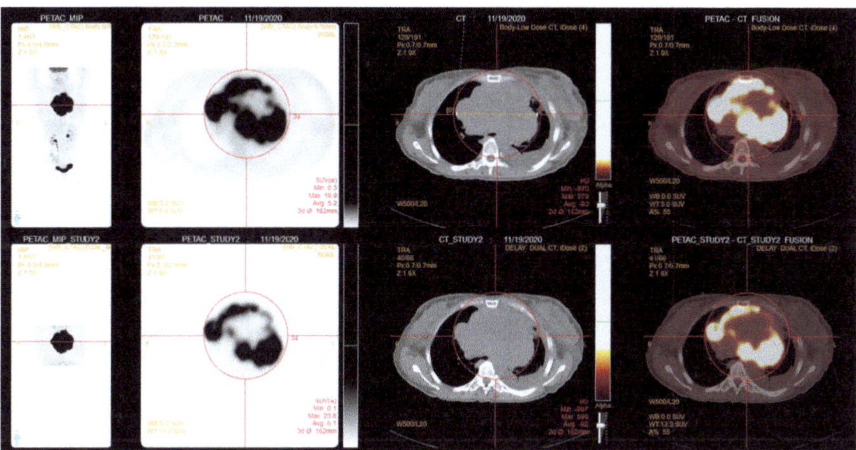

C. Y. O. Wong, D. Wu, *Phenotypic Oncology PET*,
https://doi.org/10.1007/978-3-031-09737-9_93

B: Pathology returned positive for primary mediastinal (thymic) large B-cell lymphoma, with Ki 67 of 80–90%, double-expressor phenotype (cMYC and BCL2 positive). Restaging PET-CT studies were performed during eight cycles of chemotherapy with R-EPOCH. (1) Based on the pathology and diagnostic/initial PET-CT findings, how was the prognosis? (2) How was the response to chemotherapy? (3) What were the Lugano scores? (4) What do we recommend in terms of future treatments?

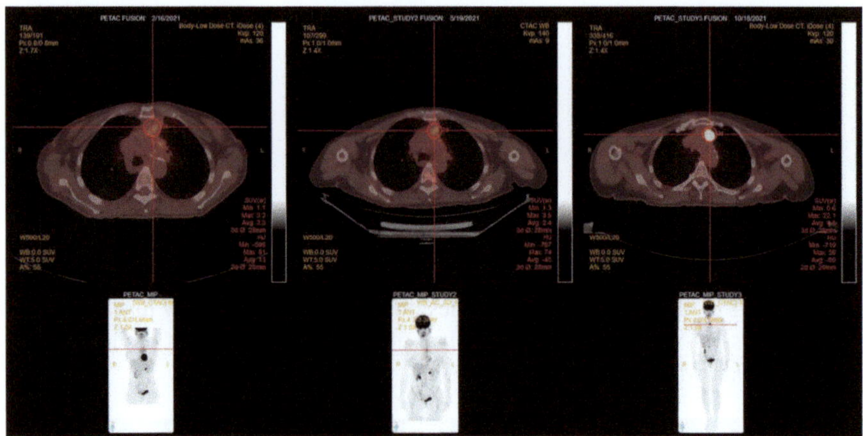

93.1 Case 93: Interpretation and Teaching

A1: F-18 FDG.

A2: Yes, the mass meets criteria for bulky mediastinal lymphoma.

A3: No, there is no appreciable FDG activity to suggest lesions other than the bulky mediastinal lymphoma.

A4: Although the FDG activity of the left pleural effusion is low (max SUV 0.8), further workup is recommended as malignant effusion cannot be excluded. Indeed, patient underwent thoracentesis and cytology positive for malignancy.

B1: The prognosis is poor, due to the pathological features and the bulky mediastinal lymphoma with a large central necrosis.

B2: As would be expected, the response to extended chemotherapy with R-EPOCH is unfavorable, with persistent FDG activity at the primary site and relapsed disease at the end (the far-right panel, dated October 18, 2021).

B3: The Lugano scores were 4–5, indicating chemo-resistance.

B4: Given the primary bulky mediastinal lymphoma at the beginning and developing chemo-resistance, consolidation radiation shall be recommended.

Teaching Point

1. According to Ann Arbor lymphoma staging system 1989, the definition for bulky mediastinal lymphoma is "the maximum width (of the lymphoma mass) is equal or greater than 1/3 of the internal transverse diameter of the thorax at the level of T5/T6."

2. In clinical practice, there is no cutoff max SUV of pleural effusions or ascites to separate malignant versus benign effusion. The case demonstrates no appreciable FDG activity (max SUV 0.8), but it cannot rule out malignant pleural effusion.

3. Bulky lymphomas are an indicator for treatment challenges and a poor prognosis, as shown in this case. Despite extended and multi-agent chemotherapy, the patient failed to achieve complete remission (CR) and eventually developed recurrent disease. Consolidation radiation therapy is indicated or shall be planned in all patients with bulky lymphomas unless otherwise contraindicated.

References

Hoppe RT. The management of bulky mediastinal Hodgkin's disease. Hematol Oncol Clin North Am. 1898;3(2):265–76.

Martelli M, Ferreri AJ, Agostinelli C, et al. Diffuse large B-cell lymphoma. Crit Rev. Oncol Hematol. 2013;87(2):146–71.

Chapter 94
Case 94: Pulmonary Sarcoid and Lung Cancer

A: Restaging PET-CT in a 72-year-old female with history of stage IIIA left lower lobe (LUL) lung adenocarcinoma treated with concurrent chemoradiation with remission. Serial CT scans show progressive tubular nodular densities in LUL, with mass-like appearance in the peripheral lung. (1) What is the tracer? (2) What is PET-CT impression and what do we recommend? (3) Moderate tracer activity is noted in the right vocal cord, but no appreciable activity on the left side. What does this indicate?

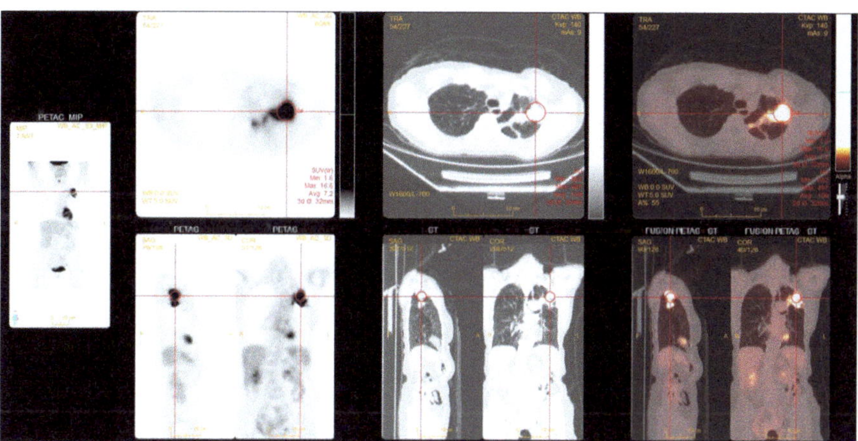

C. Y. O. Wong, D. Wu, *Phenotypic Oncology PET*,
https://doi.org/10.1007/978-3-031-09737-9_94

B: Follow-up PET-CT (using a diagnostic dual-time protocol, the left panel) showed improvement in the LUL mass-like lesion but a new nodule in the supero-lateral right lower lobe (RLL) with stable tracer intensity on delayed PET imaging. (1) What's the impression about the known LUL mass-like lesion? (2) What do we recommend with respect to the new RLL nodule?

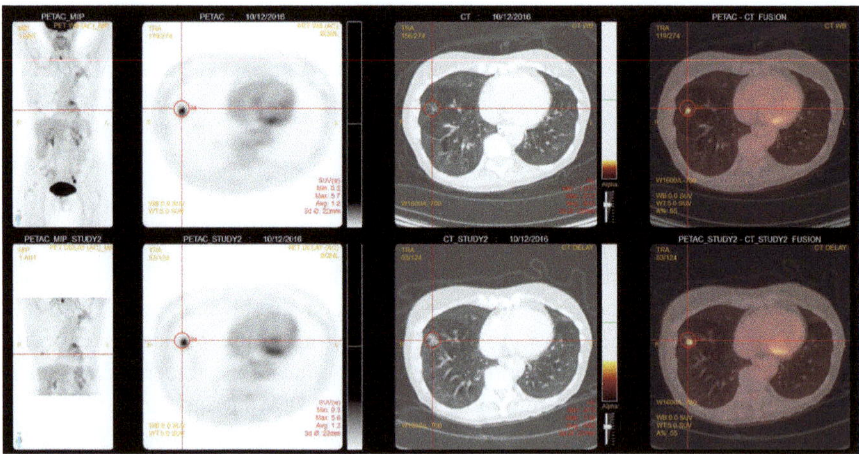

94.1 Case 94: Interpretation and Teaching

A1:   F-18 FDG.

A2:   The PET-CT is abnormal and shows heterogeneous FDG activity in the tubular nodular densities, more prominent or intense in the peripheral mass-like lesion, max SUV 16.6, concerning recurrent lung cancer versus post-radiation inflammatory changes. Therefore, further workup including biopsy for definite diagnosis is recommended.

A3:   The one-sided vocal cord FDG activity is a frequent incidental FDG PET-CT finding, often indicating vocal cord paralysis on the contralateral side, likely secondary to impaired recurrent laryngeal nerve due to tumor invasion or posttreatment injury.

B1:   The known LUL mass-like lesion shows interval decreased FDG activity, indicating improvement, consistent with biopsy-proven granuloma.

B2:   The new RLL nodule, despite the lack of enhanced activity on delayed PET imaging, is suspicious for malignancy or metastasis, for which biopsy or surgical resection for definite diagnosis is recommended.

 C: Biopsy of the RLL nodule was nondiagnostic, but patient underwent stereotactic body radiation therapy (SBRT) for the treatment of presumed RLL malignancy. Follow-up PET-CT scans were performed as the following:

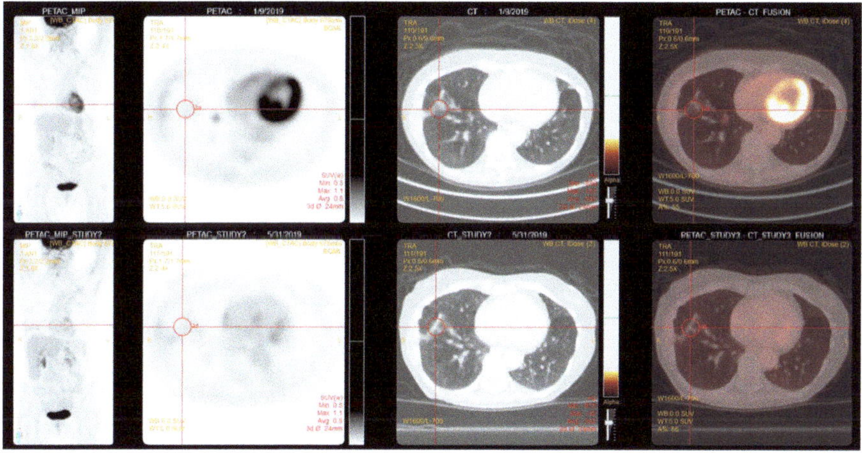

Teaching Point Due to essentially nonspecific nature of FDG activity, there is no cutoff calculated SUV that can reliably differentiate benign versus malignant/metastatic lesions, in the lungs or any other organs. This case demonstrates that active post-radiation granuloma can have as high as max SUV 16.6. On the other hand, pulmonary carcinoid tumors or adenocarcinomas with lepidic growth pattern (formerly referred as bronchoalveolar carcinoma) could have very low FDG activity with SUV < 1.0. Biopsy for definite diagnosis shall be recommended whenever there is any uncertainty.

References

Akaike G, Itani M, Shah H, et al. PET/CT in the diagnosis and workup of sarcoidosis: focus on atypical manifestations. Radiographics. 2018;38(5):1536–49.

Huang SC. Anatomy of SUV. Standardized uptake value Nucl Med Biol. 2000;27(7):643–6.

Chapter 95
Case 95: Oligo or Multiple Bone Metastasis in Newly Diagnosed Prostate Cancer?

A: Restaging PET CT in a 66-year-old male patient with newly diagnosed prostate carcinoma, without surgery, prior chemotherapy, or radiation. FDG PET-CT showed findings suspicious for bone metastases involving the right proximal femoral shaft and portion of the right ischium (data not shown). Further PET-CT using a different tracer for workup is requested before radiation therapy. (1) What is the tracer? (2) What's the impression about the prostate gland? (3) Did the patient have oligo or multiple bone metastases? (4) Is there any evidence of lymphonodal involvement?

© The Author(s), under exclusive license to Springer Nature Switzerland AG 2022

C. Y. O. Wong, D. Wu, *Phenotypic Oncology PET*,
https://doi.org/10.1007/978-3-031-09737-9_95

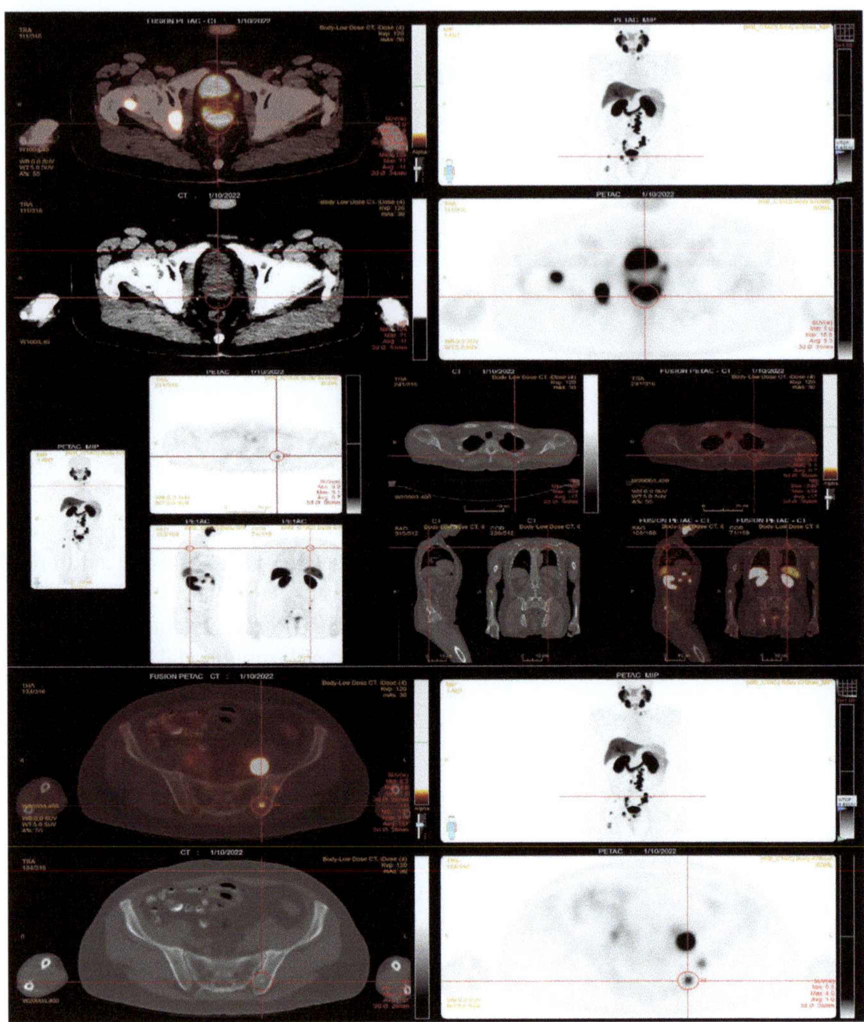

95.1 Case 95: Interpretation and Teaching

A1: F-18 PSMA (PYLarify).

A2: There is focal and intense tracer uptake within the prostate gland, more prominent in the posterior portion, consistent with known newly diagnosed prostate adenocarcinoma.

A3: In addition to multifocal abnormal tracer activity consistent with known metastases involving the right proximal femoral shaft and portion of the right ischium as demonstrated on FDG PET-CT, there are multiple foci of mild to moderate tracer activity corresponding to sclerotic changes on the concurrent CT, involving at least two right ribs (the middle panel), the L3 and L5 vertebrae, and the left iliac bone (the lower panel), highly suggestive of multiple bone metastases.

A4: Yes, there is adenopathy with variable tracer uptake, involving at least the left supraclavicular region (likely Virchow's nodes), the bilateral retroperitoneal chain, left greater than right, and the left pelvis (the lower panel), highly suggestive of extensive lymph node metastases above and below the diaphragm.

Teaching Point F-18 PSMA (PYLarify) is a new PET tracer that has been recently approved by the US FDA for imaging suspected metastatic or recurrent prostate cancer. PSMA is a protein overexpressed on the surface of more than 90% of primary and metastatic prostate carcinoma cells. As would be expected, focal intense tracer uptake is identified in the posterior portion of the prostate gland, consistent with known primary prostate cancer. Since a recent FDG PET-CT showed oligo bone metastases confined to the right proximal femur and portion of the right ischium, F-18 PSMA PET-CT was requested for further evaluation for radiation planning. This new PET imaging study clearly demonstrates multiple bone metastases, most likely leading to changes in clinical treatment planning. In addition to bone metastases, there are extensive lymphonodal metastases above and below the diaphragm, which were not appreciated on the FDG PET-CT study.

References

Pianou NK, Stavrou PZ, Vlontzou E, et al. More advantages in detecting bone and soft tissue metastases from prostate cancer using (18)F-PSMA PET CT. Hell J Nucl Med. 2019;22(1):6–9.

Rowe SP, Macura KJ, Mena E, et al. PSMA-based [18F]DCFPyL PET CT is superior to conventional imaging for lesion detection in patients with metastatic prostate cancer. Mol Imaging Biol. 2016;18(3):411–9.

Chapter 96
Case 96: Reactive Nodes and Granulomas Associated with Breast Implant Rupture

A: Restaging PET CT in a 64-year-old female with history of recurrent right breast invasive ductal carcinoma and biopsy proven right axillar nodal metastases, treated with modified right radical mastectomy, reconstruction with bilateral breast implants, completed chemotherapy and radiation. Patient experienced left breast implant rupture, status post repair one and a half years ago. (1) What is tracer? (2) Is there any evidence of recurrent or metastatic disease in the right chest? (3) What is the likely cause of the left internal mammary nodes?

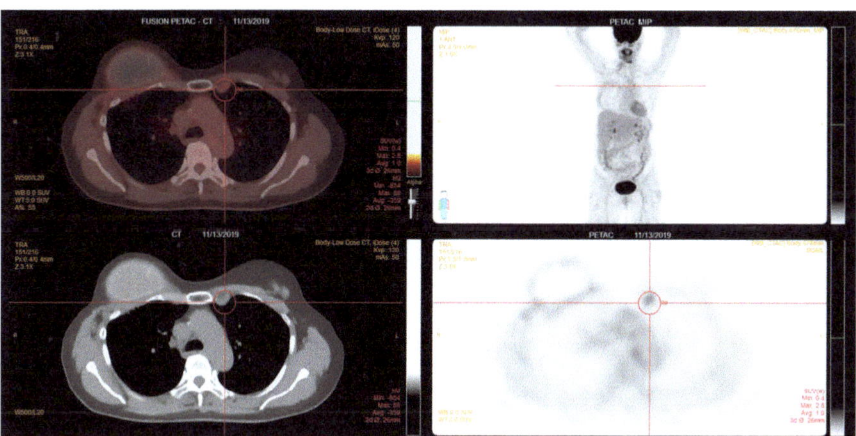

C. Y. O. Wong, D. Wu, *Phenotypic Oncology PET*,
https://doi.org/10.1007/978-3-031-09737-9_96

B: Patient had bilateral breast implants removed with bilateral capsulectomy. Surveillance FDG PET-CT was performed with images as the following: (1) What is impression about the representative left internal mammary node? (2) What does the largely symmetric pattern of numerous FDG-avid lesions in the bilateral mediastinum and hila suggest? (3) What shall we recommend?

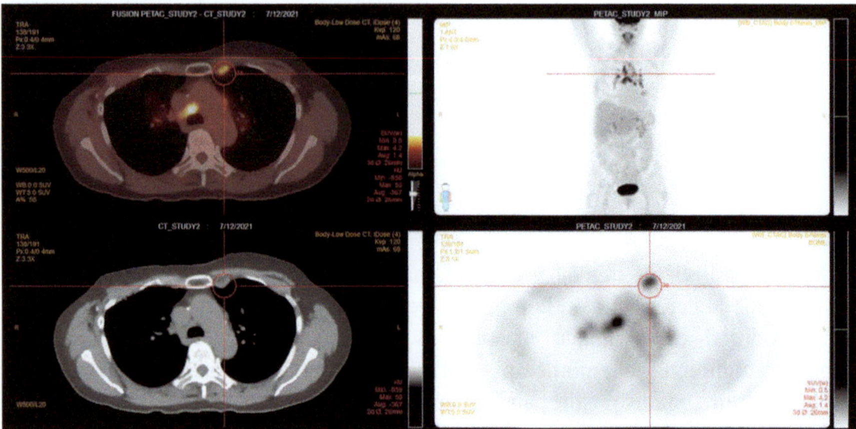

96.1 Case 96: Interpretation and Teaching

A1: F-18 FDG.

A2: No, the known right breast implant is in place, without discrete abnormal FDG activity at the interface. Imaging of the right axillary region is also unremarkable.

A3: On the left, however, there are prominent or enlarged internal mammary nodes with minimal to mild FDG activity. The largest one as shown within circle of the crosshair measures approximately 1.6 × 0.9 cm, with max SUV 2.8. There are two reasons to suggest reactive nodes instead of metastases: history of left breast implant rupture and a lack of evidence of recurrent or metastatic disease in the right chest.

B1: The largest left internal mammary node is reduced in size on CT, now measuring 1.5 × 0.6 cm, but with interval increased FDG intensity, current max SUV 4.2 in comparison to the prior SUV 2.8. The findings are still consistent with a reactive node with fluctuating metabolic activity.

B2: The overall symmetric pattern is suggestive of granulomas, although underlying metastasis cannot be excluded.

B3: Biopsy for definite diagnosis is recommended if clinically warranted. Indeed, the patient underwent FNA of station 4R and 11 L one month after the FDG PET-CT scan; both returned negative for malignancy or metastasis.

Teaching Point Breast implant rupture inevitably causes inflammation leading to the development of reactive lymph nodes that could mimic metastasis. Knowing the history of implant rupture and prior primary/metastatic sites is helpful to make a judgmental call for reactive nodes, although atypical metastasis cannot be excluded. It is well known that silicone is associated with the development of granulomas. The involvement of bilateral mediastinum and hila often exhibits a largely symmetric pattern. That has been said; asymmetric/atypical granulomas can occur, often posing challenges in the differential diagnosis of malignancy/metastasis versus active granulomas. Biopsy of representative lesions may yield definite diagnosis. Imaging follow-up to establish interval stability is a noninvasive option if clinically appropriate.

References

Naur TMH, Bodtger U, Nessar R, et al. Asymptomatic silicon induced granulomatous disease diagnosed by endobronchial ultrasound with real-time guided transbronchial needle aspiration (EBUS-TBNA). Respir Med Case Rep. 2020;30:101–2.

Palot Manzil FF, Bhambhvani PG. (18) F-FDG PET/CT unveiling of implant rupture and clinically unsuspected silicone granuloma in treated breast cancer. J Nucl Med Technol. 2018;46(4):394–5.

Chapter 97
Case 97: Metabolic Phenotypes of Anaplastic Thyroid Carcinoma and Metastases

A: Initial staging PET-CT in a 70-year-old female with newly diagnosed anaplastic thyroid carcinoma (ATC), with squamous differentiation via biopsy of neck/thyroid mass 10 days ago. Thyroglobulin (Tg) was 0.6, with positive Tg antibody. (1) What is the tracer? (2) Is the tracer intensity of a peri-thyroid node (the lower panel) different from the thyroid mass? (3) Is there any evidence of distant metastasis? (4) Is the Tg level normal?

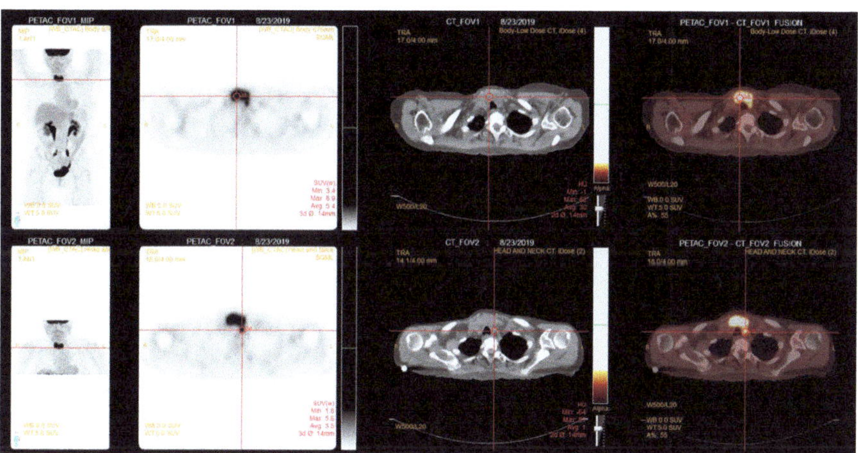

© The Author(s), under exclusive license to Springer Nature Switzerland AG 2022
C. Y. O. Wong, D. Wu, *Phenotypic Oncology PET*,
https://doi.org/10.1007/978-3-031-09737-9_97

B: After completion of neoadjuvant chemoradiation, restaging PET-CT was performed with images listed on the far-left panel. Then, patient underwent total thyroidectomy and central neck dissection with pathology confirming ATC and two nodes positive for metastasis. Restaging PET-CTs were performed with images displayed in the mid and far-right panels. Tg was <0.5, with negative Tg antibody. (1) How was the response to neoadjuvant chemoradiation? (2) Is there any of residual or metastatic disease in the post-thyroidectomy PET-CT in the mid panel? (3) What's the impression of the last PET-CT in the far-right panel?

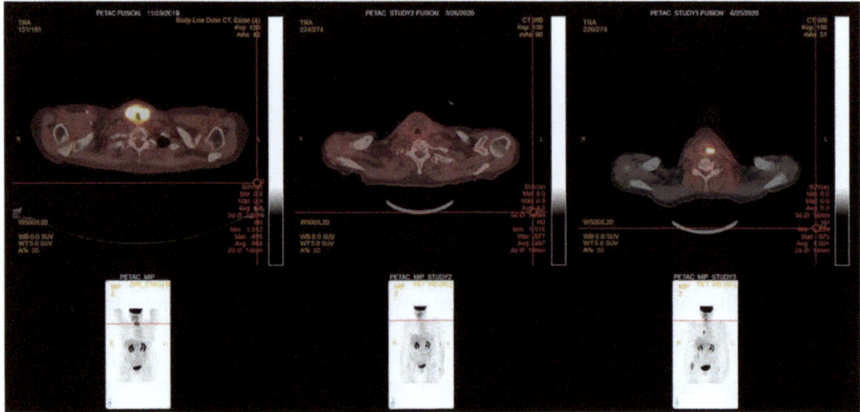

97.1   Case 97: Interpretation and Teaching

A1:   F-18 FDG.

A2:   Yes, the FDG intensity in a left peri-thyroid lymph node is near half of the main thyroid mass, indicating a different phenotypical pattern.

A3:   No, there is no discrete abnormal FDG activity to suggest distant metastasis to the chest, abdomen, or pelvis.

A4:   The thyroglobulin is falsely normal, indirect evidence of de-differentiated or anaplastic thyroid carcinoma.

B1:   The response to neoadjuvant concurrent chemoradiation was poor. The thyroid mass was interval enlarged with persistent abnormal FDG activity, now partially encasing the trachea with mass effects.

B2:   No. There is a large seroma with minimal reactive changes in the peripheral, but no evidence of FDG-avid residual or metastatic disease.

B3:   Unfortunately, the last PET-CT showed recurrent disease in the left thyroid bed and multiple foci of metastases to the right lung and hilum, which was biopsy proven to be metastatic anaplastic thyroid carcinoma with squamous differentiation.

Teaching Point   ATC is a rare primary thyroid malignancy accounting for 1–2% of all thyroid cancers. ATC is one of the most aggressive cancers in humans with a very poor prognosis. In addition to local invasion and regional lymph node metastasis, ATC has a high rate of distant metastasis, such as lung metastasis shown in this case. As would be expected, this patient had a poor response to neoadjuvant chemoradiation and surgical resection. On FDG PET, the much higher metabolic activity of the primary ATC masses relative to its metastases is in line with the tumor aggressiveness. The low levels of Tg are consistent with dedifferentiation of ATC, limiting effectiveness of RAI therapy.

References

Bogsrud TV, Karantanis D, Nathan MA, et al. 18F-FDG PET in the management of patients with anaplastic thyroid carcinoma. Thyroid. 2008;18(7):713–9.

Molinaro E, Romei C, Biagini A, et al. Anaplastic thyroid carcinoma: from clinicopathology to genetics and advanced therapies. Nat Rev. Endocrinol. 2017;13(11):644–60.

Chapter 98
Case 98: Male Breast Carcinoma

A: Initial staging PET-CT in a 65-year-old male with newly diagnosed invasive ductal carcinoma of left breast, ER and PR positive, but Her-2 negative. There is also history of benign prostate hypertrophy (BPH) but no prior history of malignancy or metastasis. (1) What is the tracer? (2) What's the impression about the known left breast cancer? (3) Is there any evidence of metastasis (locoregional or distant)? (4) How is the prognosis of primary male breast cancer? (5) What's the impression about the left kidney and ureter?

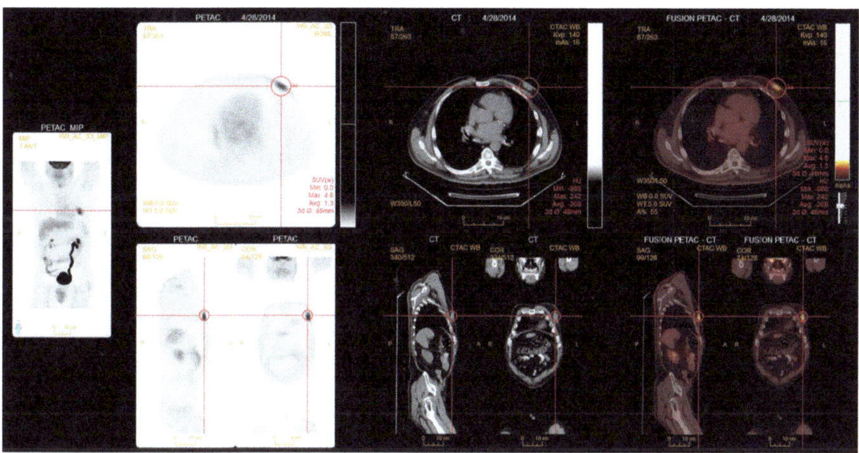

C. Y. O. Wong, D. Wu, *Phenotypic Oncology PET*,
https://doi.org/10.1007/978-3-031-09737-9_98

B: Patient was treated with neoadjuvant and concurrent chemoradiation, followed by left radical mastectomy. While on maintenance of hormone therapy, patient had serial whole-body bone scans, with selected images as the following: (1) What is the tracer? (2) How was the response to hormone therapy? (3) What's the clinical implication/significance of the worsening lesions in the left proximal femur?

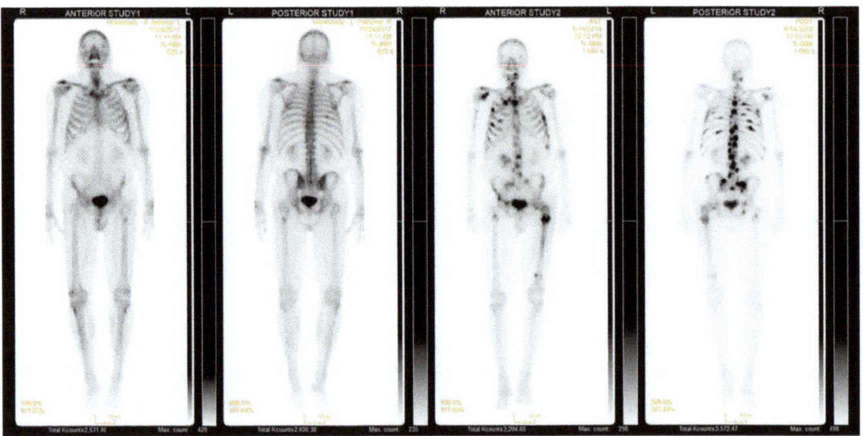

98.1   Case 98: Interpretation and Teaching

A1:   F-18 FDG.

A2:   The known left breast mass shows moderate FDG activity, max SUV 4.8, consistent with biopsy-proven breast carcinoma, with a moderate metabolic rate.

A3:   No, there is no discrete abnormal FDG activity to suggest local or distant metastasis.

A4:   Although the lack of metastasis in this case indicates early stage of disease, many patients with newly diagnosed male breast cancer present with widespread metastases at the beginning, consistent with advanced disease. No matter what is the clinical stage at diagnosis, male breast cancers often have more aggressive clinical behavior, with a poor prognosis.

A5:   The intense urine FDG activity in the dilated left renal pelvis and ureter raises concerns of obstructive hydroureteronephrosis.

B1:   Tc-99 m MDP.

B2:   The response to hormone therapy was poor, as evidenced with progression of bone metastases over years of observation. More specifically, although a baseline bone scan was negative (data not shown), follow-up bone scan (the left panel) showed bone metastases involving at least the left proximal femoral shaft, the posterior portion of the right eighth rib, and multiple levels of the thoracic spine. One and a half years later, another follow-up bone scan (the right panel) revealed widespread bone metastatic disease in the axial skeleton and the proximal appendicular skeleton, with an increasing risk for pathological fracture in the left proximal femur. CT images show newly developed or worsening metastatic disease involving at least the lungs and brain (data not shown) despite ongoing maintenance hormone therapy.

B3:   The interval worsening bone metastasis in the left proximal femoral shaft carries an increased risk for pathological fracture. Definite treatment is recommended.

Teaching Point   Male breast carcinomas are a rare malignancy but often associated with treatment failure and a poor prognosis. Most of the patients with male breast cancer present with advanced disease upon diagnosis. Although the pathological and molecular features of male breast cancers as well as treatment strategies are very similar to the females, the overall response rate and prognosis are much worse in comparison to females with breast cancers. As shown in this case, although the patient received all kinds of therapies, including neoadjuvant chemoradiation, radical mastectomy, and hormone therapy; he succumbed to metastatic breast cancer only 5 years after initial diagnosis.

References

Goss PE, Reid C, Pintilie M, et al. Male breast carcinoma: a review of 229 patients who presented to the Princess Margaret Hospital during 40 years: 1955–1996. Cancer. 1999;85(3):629–39.

Piciu A, Ficiu D, Polocoser N, et al. Diagnostic performance of F18-FDG PET/CT in male breast cancers patients. Diagnostics (Basel). 2021;11(1):119.

Chapter 99
Case 99: Advanced Hepatocellular Carcinoma (HCC) Featured by IVC/Right Atrial Tumor Thrombus

A: Initial staging PET-CT was performed in a 73-year-old male with newly diagnosed hepatic cell adenocarcinoma (HCC), well and moderate differentiated. Medical oncology history is significant for laryngeal cancer, treated with total laryngectomy, followed by concurrent chemoradiation of 12 years ago. Current AFP was 29.9 ng/mL, rising in comparison to the prior level of 5.5 ng/mL 1 month ago. (1) What is the tracer? (2) Redemonstrated is a hepatic dome mass, presumed to be biopsy-proven HCC. How was the metabolic activity of the primary mass? (3) In addition, what's the PET-CT impression about a lesion within the IVC and right atrium with mild and heterogeneous tracer activity? (4) What's the likely cause of a soft tissue lesion in the left retro-oropharyngeal wall with focal and intense tracer uptake?

C. Y. O. Wong, D. Wu, *Phenotypic Oncology PET*,
https://doi.org/10.1007/978-3-031-09737-9_99

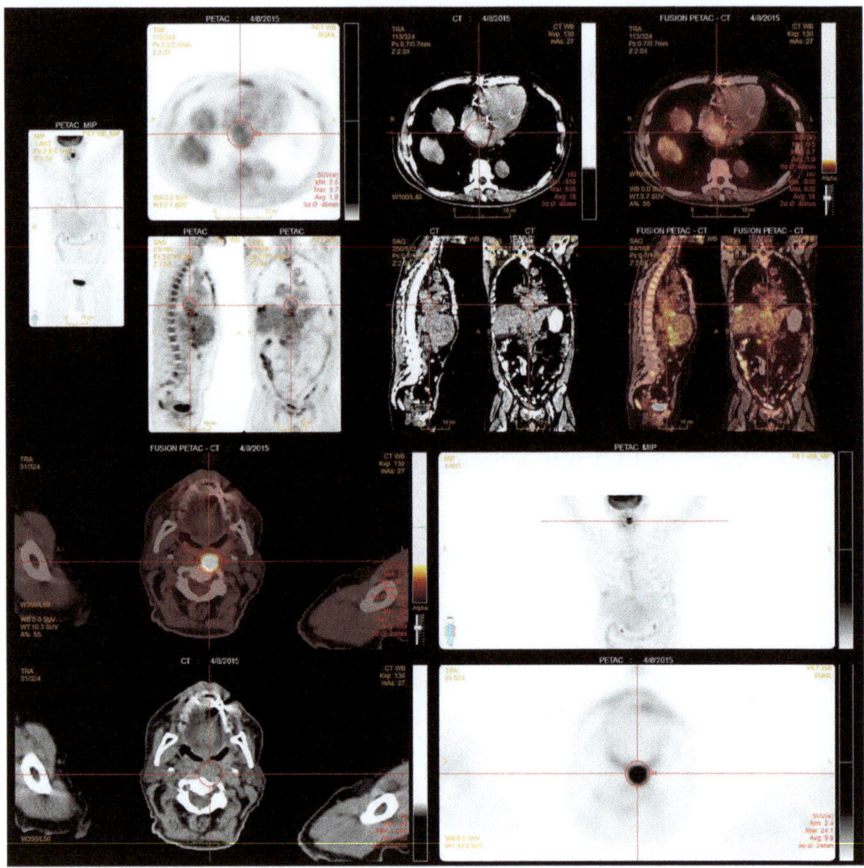

99.1 Case 99: Interpretation and Teaching

A1: F-18 FDG.

A2: The hepatic dome mass only shows mildly increased FDG activity, max SUV 4.9 in comparison to max SUV 3.2 in the surrounding normal liver parenchyma, indicating a low metabolic rate of the biopsy-proven HCC primary mass.

A3: The intrahepatic IVC is dilated, with heterogeneous appearance on the concurrent CT and heterogeneous FDG (data not shown), extended into the right atrium (circle of crosshair), suspicious for ICV/right atrium metastatic/tumor thrombus, with a mild metabolic activity. The intra-IVC/right atrium tumor thrombus is best delineated on a diagnostic/IV-contrasted CT as the following:

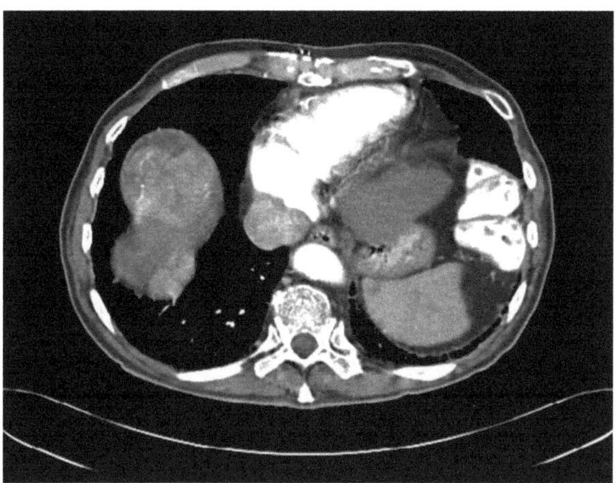

A4: Given the remote history of laryngeal cancer, the new PET CT finding of a retro-oropharyngeal mass with intense FDG activity, max SUV 24.1, is suspicious for recurrent or metastatic disease. Biopsy is recommended if warranted.

Teaching Points

1. This case illustrates a relatively low metabolic phenotype of primary HCC and its tumor thrombus withint the IVC/right atrium, probably due to persistent glucose-6-phosphatase (G6Pase) within HCC cells that converts FDG-6-P back into FDG, thus reducing intracellular trapped FDG-6-P with HCC lesions. This explains the low metabolic phenotype of HCC.
2. HCC-associated IVC/right atrial tumor thrombus is a rare condition, often associated with a very poor prognosis. This patient had an additional malignancy presenting as recurrent laryngeal cancer. Indeed, the patient died after a few months of palliative radiation therapy.

References

Kuang Y, Schomisch SJ, Chandrmouli V, Lee ZH. Hexokinase and glucose-6-phosphatase activity in woodchuck model of hepatitis virus-induced hepatocellular carcinoma. Comp Biochem Physiol C Toxicol Pharmacol. 2006;143(2):225–31.

Wolfort RM, Papillion PW, Turnage RH. Role of FDG-PET in the evaluation and staging of hepatocellular carcinoma with comparison of tumor size, AFP level, and histologic grade. Int Surg. 2010;95(1):67–75.

Xia Y, Zhang J, Ni X. Diagnosis, treatment and prognosis of hepatocellular carcinoma with inferior vena cava/right atrium tumor thrombus. Oncol Lett. 2020;20(4):101.

Chapter 100
Case 100: Metabolic Phenotype of Primary Lung Cancer-Associated Pulmonary Lymphangitic Carcinomatosis (PLC)

A: An initial PET-CT in a 58-year-old male with newly diagnosed metastatic lung adenocarcinoma, via excisional biopsy of a left supraclavicular node. (1) What is the tracer? (2) Is there any evidence for lung primary malignancy? (3) What's the impression about the findings in the right lung (at middle and lower lobes)?

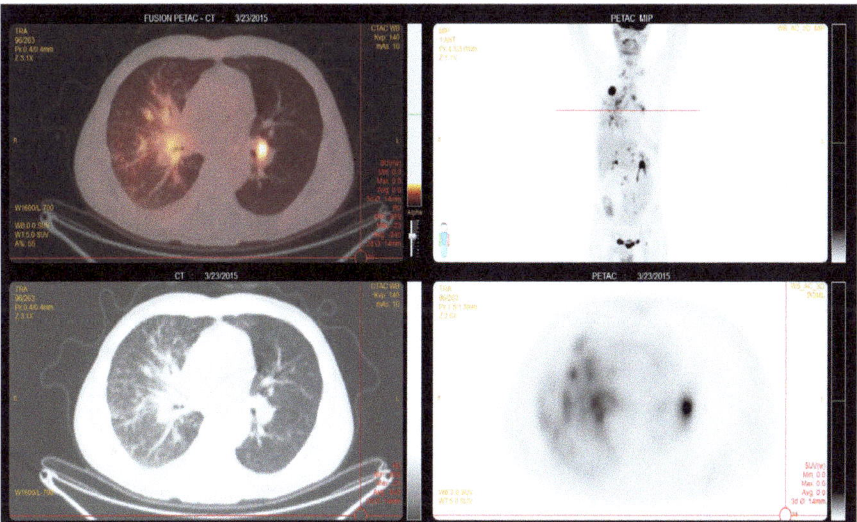

C. Y. O. Wong, D. Wu, *Phenotypic Oncology PET*,
https://doi.org/10.1007/978-3-031-09737-9_100

B: One day after the PET-CT scan, patient underwent MRI brain for further staging. (1) In the right temporal lobe, there are two subtle and small enhancing foci. What is the most likely cause?

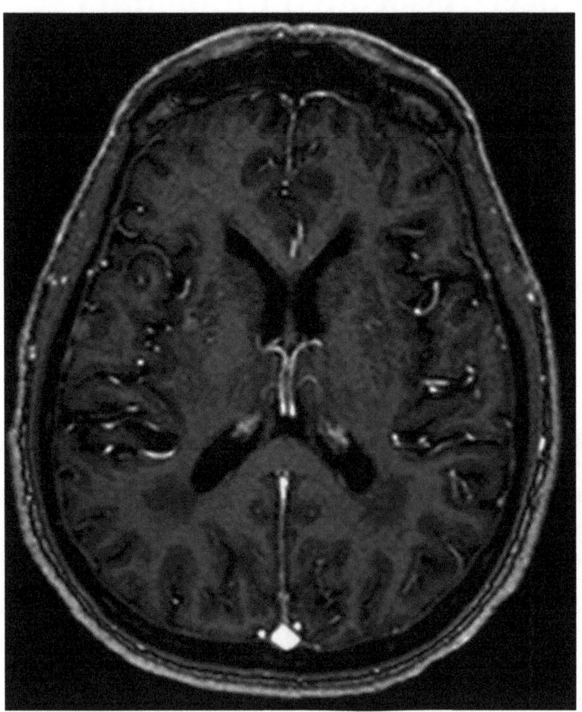

100.1   Case 100: Interpretation and Teaching

A1: F-18 FDG.
A2: Yes, there is a right upper lobe (RUL) spiculate mass in the central right upper lobe measuring approximately 3.0 × 3.5 cm, with intense FDG uptake, max SUV 13.9, suggestive of right upper lung primary malignancy with a high metabolic phenotype.
A3: In addition to lymphonodal metastases above and below the diaphragm as well as multiple sites of bone metastases, the lung window images show diffuse infiltrates with nodularity, with interlobular septal thickening, mainly involving the right middle lobe and right lower lobe (RML and RLL), showing a "dot in box" appearance, with heterogeneous FDG activity, max SUV 6.0, suspicious for right pulmonary lymphangitic carcinomatosis (PLC).
B1: Although it is subtle, the finding of contrast-enhanced foci in brain parenchyma (right temporal lobe) is suspicious for early stage of brain metastasis.

Teaching Point Pulmonary lymphangitis carcinomatosis (PLC), despite its rarity, can be caused by primary lung cancers or several non-pulmonary malignancies, such as advanced breast or colorectal cancers or renal cell carcinoma. Demonstrated in this case are typical CT features for PLC, plus PET findings highly suggestive of RUL primary malignancy, biopsy-proven lymphonodal metastases above and below the diaphragm, and multiple sites of bone metastases. Subsequently, MRI brain showed early stage of brain metastases. PLC is not only an imaging finding of significance but also an indicator for a very poor prognosis.

References

Alves C, Boavida L, Oliveira R, et al. Pulmonary lymphangitic carcinomatosis as first manifestation of cancer: case series. Chest. 2021;160(4):A1571.
Klimek M. Pulmonary lymphangitis carcinomatosis: systemic review and meta-analysis of case reports, 1970-2018. Postgrad Med. 2019;131(5):309–18.

Index